Clinical Guidelines
From Conception to Use

Clinical Guidelines
From Conception to Use

Edited by

Martin Eccles
Centre for Health Services Research
University of Newcastle upon Tyne

and

Jeremy Grimshaw
Health Services Research Unit
University of Aberdeen

Foreword by

Sir Donald Irvine
President, General Medical Council

Radcliffe Medical Press

© 2000 Martin Eccles and Jeremy Grimshaw

Radcliffe Medical Press Ltd
18 Marcham Road, Abingdon, Oxon OX14 1AA

British Library Cataloguing in Publication Data

A catalogue record for this book is available from the British Library.

ISBN 1 85775 426 3

Typeset by Acorn Bookwork, Salisbury, Wiltshire
Printed and bound by TJ International Ltd, Padstow, Cornwall

Contents

Foreword

Within the last 10 years clinical guidelines have moved into mainstream clinical medicine. Today there is a well-established body of knowledge and expertise on guideline construction. Moreover, in the United Kingdom the professional and governmental contributions to evidence-based clinical guidelines are coming together, in England and Wales through the recently established National Institute for Clinical Excellence, and in Scotland through the somewhat longer established SIGN collaboration between the Scottish Medical Royal Colleges and the Scottish Home & Health Department.

The creation of evidence-based clinical guidelines is one thing, their adoption and regular use by clinicians, quite another. Implementation is now seen as an increasingly important aspect of the development work. We already know much about the kind of aids to implementation that work best. For example, active feedback is more likely to lead to changes in practice than passive feedback. Nevertheless, there is still an unresolved problem. We know very little about the psychodynamics involved in assimilating new evidence into clinical decision making in ways that actually change behaviour. Equally, we know very little about the interactions between clinicians when, working in the same team, they collectively review their personal practice against clinical guidelines and policies they have adopted and are committed to. Change in practice does not always follow even though considered appropriate. This fact may help to account for, if not to explain, why in so many published and unpublished clinical audit studies the audit loop has not been closed.

This book, by a distinguished panel of contributors, brings together what we know about clinical guidelines and their use today. In a field that is developing so rapidly, it is good to have an authoritative statement of the art by acknowledged leaders.

I have no doubt that the forward movement will continue with increasing momentum. The medical profession's own drive to improve the consistency and reliability of clinical decision making, the public expectation that this will be done against up-to-date standards, and the enabling framework that will be provided by revalidation and clinical governance, together constitute a powerful force for positive change.

It may be truly said that the clinical guideline has now come of age as an established tool of modern medicine.

Sir Donald Irvine
January 2000

List of contributors

Martin Eccles
Centre For Health Services Research
University of Newcastle upon Tyne

Gene Feder
Department of General Practice and Primary Care
St Bartholomew's and The Royal Queen Mary and Westfield College

Chris Griffiths
Department of General Practice and Primary Care
St Bartholomew's and The Royal Queen Mary and Westfield College

Jeremy Grimshaw
Health Services Research Unit
University of Aberdeen

Richard Grol
Center for Quality of Care Research
Universities of Nijmegen and Maastricht

Brian Hurwitz
Department of Primary Care and General Practice
Imperial College School of Medicine at St Mary's

Allen Hutchinson
School of Health and Related Research
University of Sheffield

Paul Shekelle
West Los Angeles Veterans Affairs Medical Center
Los Angeles

Steven Woolf
Medical College of Virginia
Virginia Commonwealth University

Acknowledgements

The Health Services Research Unit is funded by the Chief Scientist Office of the Scottish Executive Health Department. However, the views expressed in this book are those of the authors and not the funding body.

The articles on which these chapters are based first appeared in the *British Medical Journal* and are reproduced by permission of the BMJ Publishing Group.

Introduction

Over the last 10 years, clinical guidelines have increasingly become a familiar part of medicine. Every day, clinical decisions at the bedside, rules of operation at hospitals and clinics, and health spending by governments and insurers are being influenced by guidelines. As defined by the Institute of Medicine, clinical guidelines are 'systematically developed statements to assist practitioner and patient decisions about appropriate healthcare for specific clinical circumstances'.[1] They may offer concise instructions on which diagnostic or screening tests to order, how to provide medical or surgical services, how long to hospitalise patients, or other details of clinical practice.

As guidelines diffuse into medicine, there are important lessons to learn from the first-hand experience of those who develop, evaluate and use them.[2] This book aims to reflect on these lessons. The broad interest in clinical guidelines has its origin in issues that most healthcare systems face: rising healthcare costs, fuelled by increased demand for care, more expensive technologies, and an ageing population; variations in service delivery among providers, hospitals and geographic regions and the presumption that at least some of this variation stems from inappropriate care, either over- or under-use of services; and the intrinsic desire of health-care professionals to offer, and patients to receive the best care possible. Clinicians, policy makers and payers see guidelines as a tool for making care more consistent and efficient and for closing the gap between what clinicians do and what scientific evidence supports. The potential benefits and harms of clinical guidelines and an overview of their use around the world are considered in the first two chapters.

Discerning users of clinical guidelines scrutinise the methods by which they are developed.[3,4] Guideline development groups that do not follow a systematic methodology tend to recommend what a consensus of experts *believe* is good for patients, not necessarily what the evidence supports. Such opinion-based methods, although common, are more vulnerable to bias and conflicts of interest than evidence-based methods that link recommendations directly to data.[5,6] Evidence-based methods emphasise explicitness: they document the strength of the evidence (e.g. by assigning codes or other ratings), offer 'balance sheets' to quantify the potential benefits and harms of available options,[7] acknowledge when recommendations are opinion based, and clarify gaps in the evidence. The production of evidence-based clinical guidelines is expensive and time consuming. However, by their methods they should maximise validity and minimise bias (although this has not been formally tested). Methods of guideline development are discussed in Chapter 3.

Chapter 4 moves on to consider aspects of clinical practice guidelines that, in discussions about guidelines, are frequently raised as areas of concern – the legal, emotional and political aspects of clinical practice guidelines.

A fundamental problem is whether clinical guidelines developed by any means actually change practice behaviour. Simply publishing guidelines has modest, if any, effect on providers.[2,8,9] To be effective instruments for change, clinical guidelines must be coupled with active implementation strategies that promote provider acceptance (e.g. professional endorsement, educational outreach, local adaptation), provide implementation tools (e.g. standing orders, wall charts) and enable or reinforce behaviour change (e.g. computerised reminder systems, audit, feedback).[10] Methods of implementing guidelines, a subject too often ignored by those who develop clinical guidelines,[10] are explored in Chapter 5.

In the final chapter we offer a view of the way forward by discussing areas of future development – improved methods of developing clinical guidelines and improved methods of implementing them.

References

1 Field MJ and Lohr KN (eds) (1990) *Clinical Practice Guidelines: directions for a new program. Institute of Medicine, Committee to Advise the Public Health Service on Clinical Practice Guidelines.* National Academy Press, Washington, DC.

2 Field MJ and Lohr KN (eds) (1992) *Guidelines for Clinical Practice: from development to use. Institute of Medi-*

cine, Committee on Clinical Practice Guidelines. National Academy Press, Washington, DC.

3   Hayward RSA, Wilson MC, Tunis SR, Bass EB and Guyatt G (1995) Users' guide to the medical literature. VIII. How to use clinical practice guidelines. A. Are the recommendations valid? *JAMA* **274**: 570–4.

4   Cluzeau F, Littlejohn P, Grimshaw JM, Feder GS and Moran SE (1999) Development of a reliable and valid methodology for appraising the quality of clinical guidelines. *Int J Qual Ass Health Care* **11**: 21–8.

5   Woolf SH (1992) Practice guidelines: a new reality in medicine. II. Methods of developing guidelines. *Arch Intern Med* **152**: 946–52.

6   Grimshaw J and Russell I (1993) Achieving health gain through clinical guidelines. I. Developing scientifically valid guidelines. *Quality in Health Care* **2**: 243–8.

7   Eddy DM (1990) Comparing benefits and harms: the balance sheet. *JAMA* **263**: 2493, 2498, 2501.

8   Oxman AD, Thomson MA, Davis DA and Haynes RB (1995) No magic bullets: a systematic review of 102 trials of interventions to improve professional practice. *Can Med Assoc J* **153**: 1423–31.

9   Bero L, Freemantle N, Grilli R, Grimshaw JM, Harvey E and Oxman AD (eds) (1998) *The Cochrane Collaboration Review group on the effective practice and organisation of care.* Module of the Cochrane Library (CD-ROM). Update Software, Oxford.

10 Grol R (1997) Beliefs and evidence in changing clinical practice. *BMJ* **315**: 418–21.

1

The potential benefits, limitations and harms of clinical guidelines

Steven Woolf, Richard Grol, Allen Hutchinson, Martin Eccles and *Jeremy Grimshaw*

Introduction

The unbridled enthusiasm for guidelines, and the unrealistic expectations about what they will accomplish, frequently betray inexperience and unfamiliarity with their limitations and potential hazards. Naive consumers of guidelines accept official recommendations on face value, especially when they carry the imprimatur of prominent professional groups or government bodies. These disparate sentiments and the growing awareness of their limitations and harms have done little to stem the rapid promulgation of guidelines around the world. It is therefore appropriate to begin a book on clinical guidelines by considering their potential benefits and harms.

Potential benefits of clinical practice guidelines

The principal benefit of guidelines is to improve the quality of care received by patients. Whilst it is clear that in the context of rigorous evaluations clinical practice guidelines can improve the quality of patient care,[1,2] whether they achieve this in daily practice is less clear. This is partly because patients, doctors, payers and managers define quality differently and partly because current evidence about the effectiveness of guidelines is incomplete.

Potential benefits for patients

For patients (and most other people in healthcare), the greatest benefit to be achieved by guidelines is to improve health outcomes. Guidelines which promote interventions of proven benefit and discourage ineffective ones have the potential to improve morbidity, mortality and quality of life, at least for some conditions. Guidelines can also improve the consistency of care; studies around the world show that the frequency with which procedures are performed varies dramatically among doctors, specialties and geographic regions, even after controlling for case mix.[3] Patients with identical clinical problems receive different care depending on their clinician, hospital or locale. Guidelines offer a remedy, making it more likely that patients will be cared for in the same manner, regardless of where or by whom they are treated.

Clinical guidelines offer patients other benefits. Those accompanied by 'consumer' versions (lay language leaflets, audiotapes or videos) or publicised in magazines, news reports and Internet sites inform patients and the public about what their clinicians should be doing. Increasingly lay guidelines summarise the benefits and harms of available options, along with estimates of the probability or magnitude of potential outcomes.[4] Such guidelines empower patients to make more informed healthcare choices and to consider their personal needs and preferences in selecting the best option. Indeed, clinicians may first learn about new guidelines (or be reminded of oversights) when patients inquire about recommendations or treatment options.

Finally, clinical guidelines can help patients by influencing public policy. Guidelines call attention to under-recognised health problems, clinical services and preventive interventions, and to neglected patient populations and high-risk groups. Services that were not previously offered to patients may be made available as a response to newly released guidelines. Clinical guidelines developed with attention to the public good can promote distributive justice, advocating better delivery of services to those in need. In a cash-limited healthcare system, guidelines that improve the efficiency of healthcare free up resources needed for other (more equitably distributed) healthcare services.

Potential benefits for healthcare professionals

Clinical guidelines can improve the quality of clinical decisions. They offer explicit recommendations for clinicians who are uncertain about how to proceed, overturn the beliefs of doctors accustomed to outdated practices, improve the consistency of care, and provide authoritative recommendations that reassure practitioners about the appropriateness of their treatment policies. Guidelines based on a critical appraisal of scientific evidence (evidence-based guidelines) clarify which interventions are of proven benefit and document the quality of the supporting data. They alert clinicians to interventions unsupported by good science; reinforce the importance and methods of critical appraisal; and call attention to ineffective, dangerous and wasteful practices.

Clinical guidelines can support quality improvement activities. The first step in designing quality assessment tools (e.g. standing orders, reminder systems, critical care pathways, algorithms, audits) is to reach agreement on how patients should be treated, often by developing a guideline. Guidelines are a common point of reference for prospective and retrospective audits of clinician or hospital practices: the tests, therapies and treatment goals recommended in guidelines provide ready process measures (review criteria) for rating compliance with best care practices.[5]

Medical researchers benefit from the spotlight that evidence-based guidelines shine on gaps in the evidence. The methods of guideline development which feature systematic reviews focus attention on key research questions that must be answered to establish the effectiveness of an intervention[6] and highlight gaps in the identified literature. Critical appraisal of the evidence identifies design flaws in existing studies. Identifying the presence and absence of evidence can redirect the work of investigators and encourage funding agencies to support studies that fulfil this effectiveness-based agenda.

Finally, there are some uses of clinical guidelines that straddle the boundary between benefits and harms. Clinicians may seek secular (and even self-serving) benefits from guidelines. In some healthcare systems, guidelines prompt government or private payers to provide coverage or physician reimbursement for services. Specialties engaged in 'turf wars' to gain ownership over specific procedures or treatments may publish a guideline to affirm their role. Clinicians may turn to guidelines for medico-legal protection or to reinforce their position in dealing with administrators who disagree with their practice policies.

Potential benefits for healthcare systems

Healthcare systems which provide services, and government bodies and private insurers who pay for them, have found clinical guidelines potentially effective in improving efficiency (often by standardising care) and optimising value for money.[7] Implementation of certain guidelines reduces outlays for hospitalisation, prescription drugs, surgery and other procedures. Publicising adherence to guidelines may also improve public image, sending messages of commitment to excellence and quality. Such messages can promote goodwill, political support, and (in some healthcare systems) revenue. Many believe that the economic motive behind clinical guidelines is the principal reason for their popularity.

Potential limitations and harms of guidelines

The most important limitation of guidelines is that the recommendations may be wrong (or at least wrong for individual patients). Setting aside human considerations, such as inadvertent oversights by busy or weary guideline group members, guideline developers may err in determining what is best for patients for three important reasons.

First, scientific evidence about what to recommend is often lacking, misleading or misinterpreted. Only a small subset of what is done in medicine has been tested in appropriate, well-designed studies. Where studies do exist, the findings may be misleading because of design flaws which contribute to bias or poor generalisability. Guideline development groups often lack the time, resources and skills to gather and scrutinise every last piece of evidence. Even when the data are certain, recommendations for or against interventions will involve subjective value judgements when weighing the benefits against the harms. The value judgement made by a guideline development group may be the wrong choice for individual patients.

Second, recommendations are influenced by the opinions and clinical experience and composition of the guideline development group. Tests and treatments that experts *believe* are good for patients may in practice be inferior to other options, ineffective or even harmful. The beliefs to which experts subscribe, often in the face of conflicting data, can fall victim to misconceptions and personal recollections that misrepresent population norms.[8]

Third, patients' needs may not be the only priority in making recommendations. Practices which are sub-optimal from the patient's perspective may be recommended to help control costs, serve societal needs or protect special interests (e.g. physicians, risk managers, politicians).

The promotion of flawed guidelines by practices, payers or healthcare systems can encourage, if not institutionalise, the delivery of ineffective, harmful or wasteful interventions. The same parties that stand to benefit from guidelines (patients, healthcare professionals, the healthcare system) may all be harmed.

Potential harm to patients

Patients are most endangered by flawed clinical guidelines. Recommendations which do not take due account of the evidence can result in sub-optimal, ineffective or harmful practices which, if followed, deny patients their best care. Inflexible guidelines can harm by leaving insufficient room for clinicians to tailor-make care for patients' personal circumstances and medical history. What is best for patients overall, as recommended in guidelines, may be inappropriate for individuals; blanket recommendations, rather than a menu of options or recommendations for shared decision making, ignore patient preferences.[9] Thus the frequently touted benefit of clinical guidelines – more consistent practice patterns and reduced variation – may come at the expense of reducing individualised care for patients with special needs. Lay versions of guidelines, if improperly constructed and worded, may mislead or confuse patients and disrupt the doctor–patient relationship.

Clinical guidelines can affect adversely public policy for patients. Recommendations against an intervention may lead providers to drop access to or coverage for services. Imprudent recommendations for costly interventions may displace limited resources needed for other services of greater value to patients. The tendency of guidelines to focus attention on specific health issues is subject to misuse by proponents and advocacy groups, giving the public (and health professionals) the wrong impression about the relative importance of diseases and effectiveness of interventions.

Potential harm to healthcare professionals

Flawed clinical guidelines harm practitioners by providing inaccurate scientific information and clinical advice, thereby compromising the quality of care. They may encourage ineffective, harmful or wasteful interventions. Even when guidelines are correct, clinicians often find them inconvenient and time consuming to use. Conflicting guidelines from different professional bodies can also confuse and frustrate practitioners.[10] Outdated recommendations may perpetuate outmoded practices and technologies.

Clinical guidelines can also hurt clinicians professionally. Auditors and managers may unfairly judge the quality of care based on criteria from invalid guidelines. The well-intentioned effort to make guidelines explicit and practical encourages the injudicious use of certain words (e.g. 'should' versus 'may'), arbitrary numbers (e.g. months of treatment, interval between screening tests), and simplistic algorithms when supporting evidence may be lacking. Algorithms that reduce patient care into a sequence of binary ('yes/no') decisions often do injustice to the complexity of medicine and the parallel and iterative thought processes inherent in clinical judgement. Words, numbers and simplistic algorithms can be used by those who judge clinicians to unfairly repudiate those who, for legitimate reasons, follow different practice policies. Guidelines carry economic implications. Referral guidelines can shift patients from one specialty to another. A negative (or neutral) recommendation may prompt providers to withdraw availability or coverage. A theoretical concern is that clinicians may be sued for not adhering to guidelines although, as discussed in Chapter 4 in this book, this has not yet become a significant reality.

Guidelines can harm medical investigators and scientific progress if further research is inappropriately discouraged. Guidelines which conclude that a procedure or treatment lacks evidence of benefit may be misinterpreted by funding bodies as grounds for not investing in further research and for not supporting efforts to refine previously ineffective technologies.

Potential harm to healthcare systems

Healthcare systems and payers may be harmed by guidelines if following them escalates utilisation, compromises operating efficiency and/or wastes limited resources. Some clinical guidelines, especially those developed by medical and other groups unconcerned about financing, may advocate costly interventions that are unaffordable or that cut into resources needed for more effective services.

Conclusion

In the face of these mixed consequences, attitudes about whether clinical guidelines are good or bad for medicine vary from one group to another. Guidelines produced by government or payers to control spiralling costs may constitute responsible public policy, but may be resented by clinicians and patients as an invasion of personal autonomy. Guidelines developed by specialists may seem self-serving, biased and threatening to generalists. To specialists, guidelines developed without their input suffer from inadequate content expertise. Inflexible guidelines with rigid rules about what is appropriate are popular with managers, quality auditors and lawyers but are decried as 'cookbook medicine' by physicians faced with non-uniform clinical problems, and as invalid by those who cite the lack of supporting data.

Clinical guidelines are only one option for improving the quality of care. Too often, advocates view guidelines as a 'magic bullet' for healthcare problems and ignore more effective solutions. Clinical guidelines make sense when practitioners are unclear about appropriate practice and when scientific evidence can provide an answer. They are a poor remedy in other settings.

References

1 Grimshaw JM and Russell IT (1993) Effect of clinical

guidelines on medical practice: a systematic review of rigorous evaluations. *Lancet* **342**: 1317–22.

2 Effective Health Care (1994) Implementing clinical practice guidelines. **Bulletin 8**.

3 Chassin MR, Brook RH, Park RE *et al.* (1986) Variations in the use of medical and surgical services by the Medicare population. *NEJM* **314**: 285–90.

4 Entwistle VA, Watt IS, Davis H, Dickson R, Pickard D and Rosser J (1998) Developing information materials to present the findings of technology assessments to consumers: the experience of the NHS Centre for Reviews and Dissemination. *Int J Tech Assess Health Care* **14**: 47–70.

5 Agency for Healthcare Policy and Research (1995) *Using Clinical Practice Guidelines to Evaluate Quality of Care. Volume 1: Issues.* US Dept of Health and Human Services, Public Health Services, Rockville, MD.

6 Cook DJ, Mulrow CD and Haynes RB (1997) Systematic reviews: synthesis of best evidence for clinical practice. *Ann Intern Med* **126**: 376–80.

7 Shapiro DW, Lasker RD, Bindman AB and Lee PR (1993) Containing costs while improving quality of care: the role of profiling and practice guidelines. *Ann Rev Public Health* **14**: 219–41.

8 Kane RL (1995) Creating practice guidelines: the dangers of over-reliance on expert judgment. *J Law Med Ethics* **23**: 62–4.

9 Woolf SH (1997) Shared decision-making: the case for letting patients decide which choice is best. *J Fam Pract* **45**: 205–8.

10 Feder G (1994) Management of mild hypertension: which guidelines to follow? *BMJ* **308**: 470–1.

2

An international overview

Steven Woolf, Richard Grol, Allen Hutchinson, Martin Eccles and *Jeremy Grimshaw*

Introduction

Clinical guidelines, official statements from health organisations and agencies on how best to care for medical
conditions or to perform clinical procedures are increasingly common in medicine. The ascendance of clinical
guidelines as a tool for improving the quality of care and
controlling costs is international, stimulated by rising
costs, practice variations and the presumption that at
least some of this variation stems from inappropriate
care. Clinical guideline activities are too extensive to be
cited comprehensively in one chapter. Large directories
are needed to catalogue the clinical guidelines of a single
country. This overview characterises the scope of activity
by highlighting illustrative clinical guideline pro-

grammes from selected countries, but does not pretend to describe all important work. Moreover, the listing of programmes was compiled in 1997 and therefore does not capture more recent guideline developments in several countries.

Europe

United Kingdom

Clinical guidelines have existed in England for decades, issued by the NHS, royal colleges, professional societies, audit groups and health authorities. But recent years have heightened interest in clinical guidelines as a tool for implementing healthcare based on proof of effectiveness.[1,2,3] Professional bodies, encouraged by the NHS, are producing clinical guidelines for use by providers to improve care, and by purchasers to guide contracting and commissioning decisions.[4] The NHS is now using a critical appraisal instrument[5] to determine which clinical guidelines to commend to health authorities.[4]

Although historically most British clinical guidelines have derived from consensus conferences or expert opinion, there is growing interest in moving guidelines to firmer scientific ground.[6,7] This trend, taken up by several groups,[8,9,10] is exemplified in clinical guidelines from the North of England project[11,12] and Royal College of General Practitioners[13] and in programmes to implement evidence-based clinical guidelines at community level (e.g. the King's Fund programme on Promoting Action on Clinical Effectiveness [PACE] and Framework for Appropriate Care Throughout Sheffield [FACTS]). Preparing evidence-based clinical guidelines, which begins with a synthesis of available evidence, is facilitated by high-quality systematic reviews from the NHS Centre for Reviews and Dissemination,[14] the UK Cochrane Centre,[15] and technology assessments from the NHS Research and Development Programme.[16]

Within Scotland, clinical guidelines are developed in a co-ordinated manner. The Scottish Intercollegiate Guideline Network, established in 1993 by the Conference of Royal Colleges and their Faculties in Scotland, uses a systematic multidisciplinary approach to prepare evidence-based clinical guidelines.[17] National guidelines are converted at local level into formats that encourage adoption in practice.[18]

The Netherlands

In The Netherlands, the Dutch College of General Practitioners has produced clinical guidelines since 1987, issuing more than 70 clinical guidelines at a rate of 8–10 topics per year.[19,20] A rigorous procedure involves an analysis of the scientific literature, combined with consensus discussions among ordinary general practitioners and content experts.[20,21] A systematic implementation programme follows clinical guideline development, employing various methods, e.g. specific educational packages for local continuing medical education and small group peer review, telephone cards for use in practices, facilitators to introduce clinical guidelines directly to practice teams, and publication of clinical guidelines in consumer journals.[22,23] More than 80% of Dutch family physicians are aware of clinical guidelines within a few months of publication, and an average of 70% of the recommendations are followed.[20] Updating of the clinical guidelines has begun, as well as collaboration with other medical specialty societies to develop guidelines for the primary–secondary care interface. Clinical guidelines figure prominently in Dutch health policy. In 1992, a landmark report proposed clinical guidelines as a tool for priority setting,[24] presaging a similar conclusion in New Zealand (*see* page 38).

Finland and Sweden

In Finland, national and local bodies have issued more than 700 clinical guidelines since 1989.[25] Although the structure and quality of the evidence supporting the clinical guidelines were initially limited,[26] a programme for evidence-based clinical guideline development has been started. The Finnish Medical Society, Duodecim, produces print and electronic versions of primary care clinical guidelines.[27] Physicians using the computer versions reportedly consult the system an average of three times daily and change practice behaviour in half of their consultations.[25] Clinical guidelines in Sweden appear in reports by the Swedish Council on Technology Assessment in Health Care,[28] an internationally consulted technology assessment agency, and in recommendations from other government bodies.

France

In France, the Agence Nationale de l'Accréditation et d'Évaluation en Santé (ANDEM) (previously named Agence Nationale pour le Dévelopement de l'Évaluation

Médicale), the governmental technology assessment agency, has published over 100 clinical guidelines based on consensus conferences or modified guidelines from other countries.[29,30,31] ANDEM has also developed more than 140 *références médicales*, guidelines on procedural indications for use in setting coverage policy.[31,32] The clinical guidelines are disseminated through networks of general practitioners, and their effectiveness is evaluated through local audits.[33] A collaborative network to implement cancer treatment guidelines has been highly effective.[34]

Germany, Italy and Spain

Clinical guidelines are on the rise in Germany[35] and Italy[36] where a guidelines database is being developed to support national healthcare reform.[37] In Spain, the Catalan Agency for Health Technology Assessment has begun preparing clinical guidelines and teaches methods of guideline development.[38,39] Consensus guidelines figure prominently in Catalonian healthcare reform.[40] In 1996 alone, the technology assessment agency in Madrid distributed over 10 000 copies of clinical guidelines and technology assessments.[41]

Pan-European clinical guideline programmes are also emerging. These include European Union efforts to fashion a systematic approach to technology assessment, such as the EUR-ASSESS project,[42] a seven-country collaboration to study clinical guideline implementation (Kristensen, personal communication, 1997), and the worldwide Cochrane Collaboration on Effective Practice and Organization of Care Practice.[43] A collaboration between countries to develop and standardise a 'critical appraisal' instrument for use in evaluating clinical guidelines in different countries has begun.

North America

The United States and Canada have amassed as many as 28 000 guidelines.[44] Although the Agency for Health Care Policy and Research,[45] established by the US Congress in 1989, may be the most internationally recognised source of American clinical guidelines, its portfolio of 19 clinical guidelines constitutes a small sample of the thousands of guidelines in use in the United States (AHCPR terminated its clinical guideline programme in 1996). Practice guidelines, protocols, and care pathways developed by professional societies and other groups are much more ubiquitous in American hospitals and health plans, where they are used for quality improvement and cost control.[46] Over half of Americans receive care through managed care organisations, 85% of which require adherence to clinical guidelines.[47] Many such organisations purchase commercially produced clinical guidelines that emphasise shortened lengths of stay and other resource savings.[48] Canadian healthcare is largely state funded, but a similar proportion of organisations (82%) use clinical guidelines.[49] Evidence-based centres, such as at McMaster University, are active in the critical appraisal of clinical guidelines and in developing lay versions for patients.

The massive clinical guideline industry in America has created special problems and a more mature audience for guidelines than exists in many other countries. One such problem is information overload. Directories and newsletters have become necessary to monitor the hundreds of guideline topics and sponsoring organisa-tions.[44,50–53] The AHCPR, American Medical Association, and American Association for Health Plans recently established an Internet clearinghouse for clinical guide-lines (www.guidelines.gov). National groups meet regu-larly, both in the US (e.g. American Medical Association) and Canada (e.g. National Partnership for Quality in Health and Canadian Medical Association), to co-ordi-nate clinical guideline activities.

Americans have articulated evidence-based methods in manuals and other reports.[53–58] This expertise has not always found its way into actual guidelines – most American clinical guidelines remain rooted in consensus or opinion – but certain guidelines, e.g. those of the American College of Physicians,[59] US Preventive Services Task Force,[60,61] AHCPR, and American Academy of Family Physicians[62] do reflect evidence-based proce-dures. Other reports offer 'guidelines on guidelines,' on such topics as priority setting,[63] developmental methods[64,65] use of language,[66] evaluation criteria,[67,68] legal implications,[69,70,71] translation of clinical guidelines into review instruments,[72,73] and implementa-tion.[45,64,67,74–76]

Australia

Clinical guidelines in Australia date to the late 1970s, when the state health authority began endorsing guide-line booklets,[77] and they continue on a large scale today. The proliferation of clinical guidelines has prompted closer study of their quality and impact on clinicians.[78–80] In 1995, the Quality of Care and Health Outcomes Committee of the National Health and Medical Research

Council[81] and the Australian Medical Association[78] each issued reports on improving methods of clinical guideline development. The Quality of Care and Health Outcomes Committee emphasises the need for evidence-based methods and has established working parties for future clinical guideline preparation.[82]

New Zealand

Clinical guidelines in New Zealand emanate directly from national health policy. A government committee, established in 1992 to define a core list of health services, recommended the use of clinical guidelines to define clinical indications for services rather than endorsing or denying services outright.[83,84] New Zealand's recognition of the pitfalls of rationing by exclusion, choosing instead to restrict services at the point of service through clinical guidelines, received international attention in debates about rationing.[85-87] The committee has since staged consensus conferences, producing clinical guidelines on 11 topics.[86] One clinical guideline on hypertension,[88] and a subsequent cholesterol guideline from the New Zealand National Heart Foundation,[89] broke new ground methodologically by linking recommendations to patients' absolute risk probabilities rather than to generic treatment criteria.[90]

Conclusion

As experience with clinical guidelines accumulates around the world, important lessons have been learned about their potential benefits, limitations and harms, as reviewed in the previous chapter. Chief among these is that the recommendations contained in clinical guidelines should not be accepted on face value, especially without attention to how they were developed. Further, clinical guidelines by themselves appear ineffective in changing practice behaviour or improving clinical outcomes; they must be coupled with active implementation strategies to successfully change practice. The next chapter examines more closely the methods by which clinical guidelines are developed.

References

1 NHS Executive (1996) *Promoting Clinical Effectiveness: a framework for action in and through the NHS.* NHS Executive, London.
2 Sackett DL, Rosenberg WMC, Gray JAM, Haynes RB and Richardson WS (1996) Evidence-based medicine: what it is and what it isn't. *BMJ* **312**: 71–2.
3 Gray JAM (1997) *Evidence-based Healthcare: how to make health policy and management decisions.* Churchill Livingstone, New York.
4 NHS Executive (1996) *Clinical Guidelines: using clinical guidelines to improve patient care within the NHS.* NHS Executive, London.
5 Cluzeau F, Littlejohns P, Grimshaw J and Hopkins A (1995) Appraising clinical guidelines and the development of criteria: a pilot study. *J Interprofessional Care* **9**: 227–35.
6 Grimshaw J and Russell I (1993) Achieving health gain through clinical guidelines. I. Developing scientifically valid guidelines. *Quality in Health Care* **2**: 243–8.

7 Eccles M, Clapp Z, Grimshaw JM, Adams PC, Higgins B, Purves I and Russell IT (1996) North of England evidence-based guidelines development project: methods of guideline development. *BMJ* **312**: 760–2.

8 Royal College of General Practitioners (1995) *The Development and Implementation of Clinical Guidelines: Report of the Clinical Guidelines Workgroup, Royal College of General Practitioners*. Royal College of General Practitioners, Exeter.

9 Royal College of Psychiatrists (1995) *Clinical Practice Guidelines and their Development*. Royal College of Psychiatrists, London.

10 British Medical Association (1996) *Guidance Notes for Clinical Guidelines. Clinical Audit Committee, British Medical Association*. British Medical Association, London.

11 Eccles M, Freemantle N and Mason J (1998a) Evidence-based guideline for the use of ACE-inhibitors in the primary care management of adults with symptomatic heart failure. *BMJ* **316**: 1369–75.

12 Eccles M, Clarke J, Livingston M, Freemantle N and Mason J (1998b) North of England evidence-based guidelines development project: summary version of evidence-based guideline for the primary care management of dementia. *BMJ* **317**: 802–8.

13 Waddell G, Feder G, McIntosh A, Lewis M and Hutchinson A (1996) *Low Back Pain Evidence Review*. Royal College of General Practitioners, London.

14 Sheldon TA and Melville A (1996) Providing intelligence for rational decision-making in the NHS: the NHS Centre for Reviews and Dissemination. *J Clin Effect* **1**: 1–4.

15 Chalmers I and Haynes B (1994) Reporting, updating

and correcting systematic reviews of the effects of healthcare. *BMJ* **309**: 862–5.

16 NHS Executive (1996) *Report of the NHS Health Technology Assessment Programme 1996*. NHS Executive, London.

17 Scottish Intercollegiate Guideline Network (1995) *Clinical Guidelines: criteria for appraisal for national use*. Scottish Intercollegiate Guideline Network, Edinburgh.

18 Petrie JC, Grimshaw JM and Bryson A (1995) The Scottish Intercollegiate Guidelines Network initiative: getting validated guidelines into local practice. *Health Bull* **53**: 345–8.

19 Meulenberg F, Thomas S and van der Voort H (eds) (1993) *NHG Standards. 5. Examples of Guidelines for General Practice*. Dutch College of General Practitioners, Utrecht, Netherlands.

20 Grol R, Thomas S and Roberts R (1995) Development and implementation of guidelines for family practice: lessons from the Netherlands. *J Fam Pract* **40**: 435–9.

21 Thomas S (1994) Standard setting in the Netherlands: impact of the human factor on guideline development. *Br J Gen Pract* **44**: 242–3.

22 Grol R and Lawrence M (1995) *Quality Improvement by Peer Review*. Oxford University Press, Oxford.

23 Hulscher M, Van Drenth B, van der Wouden, Mokkink H, Van Weel C and Grol R (1997) Changing preventive practice: a controlled trial on the effects of outreach visits to organise prevention of cardiovascular disease. *Quality in Health Care* **6**: 19–24.

24 Government Committee on Choices in Health Care (1992) *Choices in Healthcare*. A report by the Government Committee on Choices in Health Care. Ministry

of Welfare, Health and Cultural Affairs, Rijswijk, Netherlands.

25 Mäkelä M (1996) Do general practitioners need guidelines? *Scand J Prim Healthcare* **14**: 2–3.

26 Varoness H and Mäkelä M (1997) Practice guidelines in Finland: availability and quality. *Quality in Healthcare* **6**: 75–9.

27 Jousimaa J and Kunnamo I (1993) PDRD – a computer-based primary care decision support system. *Med Inf* **18**: 103–12.

28 SBU (1995) Reports from the Swedish Council on Technology Assessment in Health Care (SBU). *Int J Tech Assess Healthcare* **11**: 634–7.

29 Agence Nationale pour le Développement de l'Évaluation Médicale (1990) *Les Conférences de Consensus: base méthodologique pour leur réalisation en France.* Agence Nationale pour le Développement, de l'Évaluation Médicale, Paris.

30 Durieux P and Roche N (1995) Les recommendations pour la pratique clinique. Bases methodologiques et utilisations. *Annales de Medecine Interne* **146**: 438–46.

31 Maisonneuve H, Cordier H, Durocher A and Matillon Y (1997) The French clinical guidelines and medical references programme: development of 48 guidelines for private practice over a period of 18 months. *J Eval Clin Pract* **3**: 3–13.

32 Agence Nationale pour le Développement de l'Évaluation Médicale (1995) *Recommendations et Références Médicales. Vols. 1 and 2.* ANDEM, Paris.

33 Matillon Y and Goldberg J (1997) Clinical practice guidelines. *Lancet* **349**: 795–6.

34 Ray-Coquard I, Philip T, Lehmann M, Fervers B, Farsi F and Chauvin F (1997) Impact of a clinical guidelines

program for breast and colon cancer in a French cancer center. *JAMA* **278**: 1591–5.

35 Ollenschlager G and Thomeczek C (1996) Medical guidelines: definitions, goals, implementation. *Z Arztl Fortbild* **90**: 355–61.

36 Grilli R, Penna A, Zola P and Liberati A (1996) Physicians' view of practice guidelines: a survey of Italian physicians. *Soc Sci Med* **43**: 1283–7.

37 Liberati A, Favaretti C, Grilli R *et al.* (1997) *A pilot project to speed up the uptake of scientific information on the practice of health services (abstract).* Proceedings of the 13th Annual Meeting of the International Society of Technology Assessment in Health Care, 25–28 May, Barcelona, Spain.

38 Granados A and Borras JM (1994) Technology assessment in Catalonia: integrating economic appraisal. *Soc Sci Med* **38**: 1643–6.

39 Jovell AJ and Navarro-Rubio MD (1995) Guías de práctica clinica. *Formación Médica Continuada* **2**: 152–6.

40 Sánchez E, Vincente R and Medina A (1997) *Consensus process in defining health policies: the case of minimum common criteria for care in Catalonia, Spain (abstract).* Proceedings of the 13th Annual Meeting of the International Society of Technology Assessment in Health Care, 25–28 May, Barcelona, Spain.

41 Hernández Torres A, Conde Olasagasti JL, Castellote Olivito JM and Gol Freixa JM (1997) *Dissemination of reports on technology assessment in health care and clinical practice guidelines by the AETS in 1996 (abstract).* Proceedings of the 13th Annual Meeting of the International Society of Technology Assessment in Health Care, 25–28 May, Barcelona, Spain.

42 Banta HD, Werkö L, Cranovski R, Granados A, Henshall C, Jonsson E, Liberati A, Matillon Y and Sheldon

T (1997) Report from the EUR-ASSESS Project. *Int J Tech Assess Health Care* **13**: 133–340.

43 Bero LA, Grilli R, Grimshaw JM, Harvey E, Oxman AD and Thomson MA (1998) Closing the gap between research and practice: an overview of systematic reviews of interventions to promote the implementation of research findings. The Cochrane Effective Practice and Organization of Care Review Group. *BMJ* **317**: 465–-8.

44 ECRI (1995) *Healthcare Standards, 1996: Official Directory.* Plymouth Meeting, PA: ECRI, 1995.

45 Agency for Health Care Policy and Research (1994) *Clinical Practice Guideline Development.* Agency for Health Care Policy and Research, Rockville, MD.

46 Horn SD (1994) *Clinical Practice Improvement: a new technology for developing cost-effective quality health care.* Faulkner & Gray, Washington, DC.

47 Jensen GA, Morrisey MA, Gaffney S and Liston DK (1997) The new dominance of managed care: insurance trends in the 1990s. *Health Affairs* **16**: 125–36.

48 Doyle RL (1995) *Healthcare Management Guidelines.* Milliman & Robertson, Albany, NY.

49 Carter AO, Battista RN, Hodge MJ, Lewis S, Basinski A and Davis D (1995) Report on activities and attitudes of organizations active in the clinical practice guidelines field. *Can Med Assoc J* **153**: 901–7.

50 American Medical Association (1997) *Directory of Practice Parameters.* American Medical Association, Chicago.

51 Canadian Medical Association (1996) *Directory of Canadian Clinical Practice Guidelines.* Canadian Medical Association, Ottawa.

52 Faulkner & Gray Inc (1997) *The Medical Outcomes and*

Guidelines Sourcebook. Faulkner & Gray, Washington, DC.

53 Woolf SH (1991) *Manual for Clinical Practice Guideline Development*. Agency for Health Care Policy and Research, Rockville, MD.

54 Eddy DM (1992) *A Manual for Assessing Health Practices and Designing Practice Policies: the explicit approach*. American College of Physicians, Philadelphia.

55 Office of Technology Assessment (1994) *Identifying Health Technologies That Work: searching for evidence*. Office of Technology Assessment, Congress of the United States, Washington, DC.

56 McCormick KA, Moore SR and Siegel R (eds) (1995) *Clinical Practice Guideline Development: methodology perspectives*. Agency for Health Care Policy and Research, Rockville, MD.

57 Marek KD (1995) *Manual to Develop Guidelines. American Nurses Association, Committee on Nursing Practice Standards and Guidelines*. American Nurses Publications, Washington, DC.

58 Woolf SH (in press) *Manual for Conducting Systematic Reviews*. Agency for Health Care Policy and Research, Rockville, MD.

59 American College of Physicians (1995) *Clinical Practice Guidelines*. American College of Physicians, Philadelphia.

60 US Preventive Services Task Force (1996) *Guide to Clinical Preventive Services* (2e). Williams & Wilkins, Baltimore.

61 Woolf SH, DiGuiseppi CG, Atkins D and Kamerow DB (1996) Developing evidence-based clinical practice guidelines: lessons learned by the US Preventive Services Task Force. *Annu Rev Public Health* **17**: 511–38.

62 American Academy of Family Physicians (1993) *AAFP and Clinical Policies.* American Academy of Family Physicians, Kansas City, MO.

63 Field MJ (ed) (1995) *Setting Priorities for Clinical Practice Guidelines. Institute of Medicine, Committee on Methods for Setting Priorities for Guideline Development.* National Academy Press, Washington, DC.

64 Field MJ and Lohr KN (eds) (1992) *Guidelines for Clinical Practice: from development to use. Institute of Medicine, Committee on Clinical Practice Guidelines.* National Academy Press, Washington, DC.

65 Canadian Medical Association (1994) *Guidelines for Canadian Clinical Practice.* Canadian Medical Association, Ottawa.

66 Budetti P (1992) *Use of Language in Clinical Practice Guidelines.* Agency for Health Care Policy and Research, Rockville, MD.

67 Field MJ and Lohr KN (eds) (1990) *Clinical Practice Guidelines: directions for a new program. Institute of Medicine, Committee to Advise the Public Health Service on Clinical Practice Guidelines.* National Academy Press, Washington, DC.

68 American Medical Association (1997) *Attributes to Guide the Development and Evaluation of Practice Parameters/Guidelines.* American Medical Association, Chicago.

69 Jutras D (1993) Clinical practice guidelines as legal norms. *Can Med Assoc J* **148**: 905–8.

70 General Accounting Office (1994) *Medical Malpractice: Maine's use of practice guidelines to reduce costs.* US General Accounting Office, Washington, DC.

71 Ferrara K (1995) *Legal Issues Associated With the Use and Development of Practice Guidelines.* UHC Services Corporation, Oak Brook, IL.

72 Schoenbaum SC and Sundwall DN (eds) (1995) *Using Clinical Practice Guidelines to Evaluate Quality of Care.* Agency for Health Care Policy and Research, Rockville, MD.

73 Center for Clinical Quality Evaluation (1997) *AHCPR Guideline Criteria Project.* Agency for Health Care Policy and Research, Rockville, MD.

74 American Hospital Association (1992) *CPG Strategies: putting guidelines into practice.* American Hospital Association, Chicago.

75 Canadian Medical Association, Department of Health Care and Promotion (1993) Workshop on clinical practice guidelines: summary of proceedings. *Can Med Assoc J* **148**: 1459–62.

76 Carter AO, Battista RN, Hodge MJ, Lewis S and Haynes RB (1995) Proceedings of the 1994 Canadian Clinical Practice Guidelines Network Workshop. *Can Med Assoc J* **153**: 1715–19.

77 Hemming M and Mashford ML (1993) It works in Australia. *BMJ* **307**: 678.

78 Rice MS (1995) Clinical practice guidelines. *Med J Aust* **163**: 144–5.

79 Ward JE and Grieco V (1996) Why we need guidelines for guidelines: a study of the quality of clinical practice guidelines in Australia. *Med J Aust* **165**: 574–6.

80 Gupta L, Ward JE and Hayward RSA (1997) Clinical practice guidelines in general practice: a national survey of recall, attitudes and impact. *Med J Aust* **166**: 69–72.

81 National Health and Medical Research Council. Quality of Care and Health Outcomes Committee (1995) *Guidelines for the Development and Implementation of Clinical Practice Guidelines.* National Health and Medical Research Council, Canberra.

82 O'Brien PE (1996) Clinical practice guidelines. *Med J Aust* **164**: 54.

83 Cooper MH (1995) Core services and the New Zealand health reforms. *Br Med Bull* **51**: 799–807.

84 National Advisory Committee on Core Health and Disability Support Services (1994) *Third Report of the National Advisory Committee on Core Health and Disability Support Services to the Minister of Health.* National Advisory Committee on Core Health and Disability Support Services, Wellington.

85 Ham C (1995) Synthesis: what can we learn from international experience? *Br Med Bull* **51**: 819–30.

86 Honigsbaum F, Calltorp J, Ham C and Holmström S (1995) *Priority Setting Processes for Healthcare.* Radcliffe Medical Press, Oxford.

87 Klein R, Day P and Redmayne S (1996) *Managing Scarcity: priority setting and rationing in the National Health Service.* Open University Press, Buckingham.

88 National Advisory Committee on Core Health and Disability Support Services (1992) *The Management of Raised Blood Pressure in New Zealand.* National Advisory Committee on Core Health and Disability Support Services, Wellington.

89 Jackson R and Beaglehole R (1995) Evidence-based management of dyslipidaemia. *Lancet* **346**: 1440–2.

90 Jackson R and Sackett D (1996) Guidelines for managing raised blood pressure: evidence-based or evidence-burdened. *BMJ* **313**: 64–5.

3

Developing guidelines

Paul Shekelle, Steven Woolf, Martin Eccles and *Jeremy Grimshaw*

Introduction

The rationale for developing guidelines is to achieve better health outcomes for patients, or better value for money than would have been achieved in the absence of guidelines. Therefore the methods of guideline development should ensure that treating patients according to the guidelines will achieve the outcomes desired. Three issues underpin the development of valid and useable guidelines: 1) the development of guidelines requires sufficient resources both in the form of persons with a wide range of skills, including expert clinicians, health services researchers, and group process leaders and financial resources; 2) a systematic review of the

Box 3.1. Five steps in clinical practice guideline development

- identifying and refining the subject area of a guideline
- convening and running guideline development groups
- assessing the evidence about the clinical question or condition

evidence should be at the heart of every guideline; 3) the expert group assembled to translate the evidence into a guideline should be multidisciplinary.

There are five steps in the initial development of an evidence-based guideline (*see* Box 3.1): identifying and refining the subject area of a guideline; convening and running guideline development groups; assessing the evidence about the clinical question or condition; translating the evidence into a clinical practice guideline; and external review of the guideline. A guideline will also require review after an appropriate period of time. The dissemination, implementation and evaluation of practice guidelines will be discussed in Chapter 5.

Identifying and refining the subject area of a guideline

Prioritising topics for guideline development

Guidelines can be developed for a wide range of subjects. Clinical areas can be concerned with conditions (diabetes, coronary artery disease) or procedures (hysterectomy, coronary artery bypass surgery). Given the large number of potential areas, some form of prioritisation is needed to select a particular area for guideline development. Potential areas for practice guideline development can emerge from an assessment of the major causes of morbidity and mortality for a given population, uncertainty about the appropriateness of healthcare processes or the evidence that they are effective in improving patient outcomes, or the need to conserve resources in providing care.

Refining the subject area of a guideline

However, once the topic for guideline development is identified, it will usually need to be refined before beginning an assessment of the evidence in order to answer exact questions. This can be achieved in a number of ways. The usual way is by a dialogue among clinicians, patients and the potential end-users or evaluators of the guideline. Discussions about the scope of the guideline will also take place within the guideline development panel.

Failure to carry out this refinement runs the risk of leaving the clinical condition or question too broad in scope. For example, a guideline on 'the management of diabetes' could conceivably cover both primary, secondary and tertiary care elements of management and multiple aspects of management, such as screening, diagnosis, dietary management, drug therapy, risk factor management, or indications for referral to a consultant. While all of these could be legitimate areas for guideline development, such a task would be considerable; therefore a group needs to be clear which areas are and are not within the scope of their activities. It is possible to develop guidelines that are both broad in scope and evidence based, but to do so usually requires a considerable investment in both time and money, both of which are frequently underestimated by inexperienced developers of evidence-based clinical practice guidelines.

One method to both define the clinical question of interest and identify for exactly which processes evidence needs to be collected and assessed is the construction of models or causal pathways.[1] A causal pathway is a diagram that illustrates the linkages between intervention(s) of interest and the intermediate, surrogate and health outcomes that the interventions are thought to influence. In designing the pathway, guideline developers make explicit the premises on which their assumptions of effectiveness are based and the outcomes (benefits and harms) that they consider important. This identifies the specific questions that must be answered by the evidence to justify conclusions of effectiveness and highlights gaps in the evidence for which future research is needed.

Convening and running guideline development groups

Setting up a guideline development project

To successfully achieve the task of guideline development it may be necessary to convene more than one group. Potential groups would be a project or management team to undertake the day-to-day running of the work, such as the identification, synthesis and interpretation of relevant evidence, the convening and running of the guideline development groups, and the production of the resulting guidelines. Additional guideline development group(s) would undertake the task of producing the guidelines' recommendations in the light of the evidence or its absence. While there is no single right way to set up such groups, it is important to ensure that guideline development is adequately resourced, particularly as groups often report underestimating the resources required for the task – both in terms of finance and project management and general administrative support.

The guideline development group: membership and roles

The composition of a guideline development group can be considered in two ways: by the disciplines of the group members who would be stakeholders in the area of the guideline; and by the roles required within the group.

Group members
Identifying stakeholders involves identifying all the groups whose activities would be covered by the guideline or who have other legitimate reasons for having an input into the process. This is important to ensure adequate discussion of the evidence (or its absence) when developing the recommendations in the guideline. There is good evidence that when presented with the same evidence a single specialty group will reach

different conclusions from a multidisciplinary group, with the former being systematically biased in favour of performing procedures in which the specialty has a vested interest.[2,3] For example, the conclusions of a group of vascular surgeons favoured the use of carotid endarterectomy more than did a mixed group of surgeons and medical specialists.[4] There are good theoretical reasons to believe that individuals' biases are better balanced in multidisciplinary groups, and that such balance will produce more valid guidelines. Ideally the group should have at least six but no more than 12 to 15 members; too few members limits adequate discussion and too many makes effective functioning of the group difficult. Under certain circumstances (e.g. when developing guidelines for broad clinical areas) it may be necessary to trade off full representation against the requirement of having a functional group.

Roles
Potential roles required within guideline development groups are: group member; group leader; specialist resource; technical support; and administrative support. Group members, as indicated above, are invited to participate as individuals working in their field. Their role is to develop recommendations for practice based upon the available evidence and their knowledge of the practicalities of clinical practice.

The role of the group leader is both to ensure that the group functions effectively (the group process) and that it achieves its aims (the group task). Although guideline groups are often chaired by pre-eminent experts in the topic area, we believe the process is best moderated by someone familiar with (though not necessarily an expert in) the management of the clinical condition and the scientific literature, but who is not an advocate. Such an individual acts to stimulate discussion and allow the group to identify where true agreement exists, but not inject their own opinion in the process. This requires someone with both clinical skills and group process skills. There is also evidence that conducting the group meetings using formal group processes, rather than informal ones, produces different and possibly better outcomes.[5,6,7]

Guideline processes will require a variety of specialist support at various times and this may be fulfilled by more than one individual. Some of the potential skills required are shown in Box 3.2. Finally, groups will require administrative support for such tasks as preparing papers for meetings, taking notes and arranging venues.

Box 3.2.   Skills needed in guideline development

- literature searching and retrieval
- epidemiology
- biostatistics
- health services research (including health economies)
- clinical experts
- group process experts
- writing and editing.

Identifying and assessing the evidence

Identifying and assessing the evidence is best done by performing a systematic review. The purpose of a systematic review is to collect all available evidence,

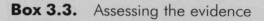

Box 3.3.   Assessing the evidence

- collect all the evidence
- assess the evidence for relevance
- assess the evidence for susceptibility to bias
- extract and summarise evidence about benefits, costs, and harms.

assess its potential applicability to the clinical question under consideration, inspect the evidence for susceptibility to bias, and extract and summarise the findings (*see* Box 3.3).

What sort of evidence?

The identification of the clinical questions of interest (using clinical pathways) will help set the boundaries for admissible evidence (the types of study designs, the year of publication, etc.). For example, questions of the efficacy of interventions usually mean that randomised-controlled trials should be sought, while questions of risk usually mean that prospective cohort studies should be sought. Similarly, studies of interventions need be searched only back until their introduction (for example, non-steroidal anti-inflammatory drugs were introduced in the early 1970s; while digoxin or digitalis has been used for over 100 years).

Where to look for evidence

The first step in gathering the evidence is to see if a suitable, recent systematic review has already been published. The Cochrane Library includes the Cochrane trials register, the database of systematic reviews and the database of abstracts of reviews of effectiveness. Relevant Cochrane review groups should also be contacted to see if a review is in progress.

Failing the availability of a current systematic review, a computerised search of Medline and Embase is the usual starting point, using search strategies that have been previously shown to be sensitive for detecting the types of studies one is looking for (though these have only been validated for randomised-controlled trials[8]). For example, randomised-controlled trials provide the best evidence to answer questions about the effectiveness of treatments, whereas prospective cohort studies provide the best evidence for questions about risk. The Cochrane trials register contains references to over 190 000 clinical trials which have been identified through database and hand searching and represents the best initial source of such studies. As such it should be examined early on in any review process. It is helpful to check the references of all the articles identified to see if there are additional relevant articles not identified by the computerised search. Having experts in the field examine the list of articles helps to ensure there are no obvious omissions. Additional search strategies, including searches for articles published in languages other than English,[9,10,11] computerised searches of specialised databases, hand searching relevant journals, and searching for unpublished material, will, in many cases, yield additional studies, but the resources needed for such activities are considerable and may not be feasible. The cost-effectiveness of various search strategies has not been established. It is best to match the scope of the search strategy to the available resources.

Assessing studies for relevance

The studies identified are then assessed for relevance to the clinical questions of interest and their susceptibility to bias. This is usually a two-step process. The initial screen or sift for relevance (often possible by reading the abstract) narrows the set to those needing a more detailed assessment. In both cases, the use of explicit rather than implicit criteria should improve the reliability of the process. There is empirical evidence that the use of two persons working independently improves the accuracy of this step in data collection.[12]

Susceptibility to bias is dependent upon study design. Randomised-controlled trials are by design less susceptible to bias than case series studies for answering questions about the efficacy of interventions;[13,14] prospective cohort studies are less susceptible to bias than retrospective cohort studies for answering questions about risk. Susceptibility to bias is also affected by the subsequent conduct of a study (e.g. studies in which randomisation is inadequately concealed are more susceptible to bias).[15] Whilst there are many different scoring systems for assessing the quality of studies, there is little empirical evidence about their validity.[16] Guideline developers should focus on methodological criteria for which there is empirical evidence of importance.

Summarising evidence

In the last step, data are extracted from the relevant studies on the benefits, harms and, where applicable, costs of the interventions being considered. These are usually presented in a form which facilitates easy comparison of the designs and results of studies. Where appropriate, meta-analysis can be used to summarise results of multiple studies.

Box 3.4. Classification scheme to grade the category of evidence supporting practice guideline statements and the strength of recommendations

Category of evidence

Ia: evidence from meta-analysis of randomised-controlled trials

Ib: evidence from at least one randomised-controlled trial

IIa: evidence from at least one controlled study without randomisation

IIb: evidence from at least one other type of quasi-experimental study

III: evidence from non-experimental descriptive studies, such as comparative studies, correlation studies and case-control studies

IV: evidence from expert committee reports or opinions and/or clinical experience of respected authorities.

Strength of recommendation

A.   directly based on Category I evidence

B.   directly based on Category II evidence or extrapolated recommendation from Category I evidence

C.   directly based on Category III evidence or extrapolated recommendation from Category I or II evidence

D.   directly based on Category IV evidence or extrapolated recommendation from Category I, II or III evidence.

Categorising evidence

Summarised evidence is categorised to reflect its under-lying susceptibility to bias. This is a shorthand method of conveying to a guideline reader specific aspects of the evidence. Several such 'strength of evidence' classifica-tion schemes exist, but empirical supporting evidence only exists for those categorising effectiveness studies.[15,16] An example of a simple scheme is shown in Box 3.4. We suggest that guideline developers should use a limited number of explicit criteria incorporating those for which there is explicit evidence.

Translating evidence into a clinical practice guideline

Evidence alone is not sufficient to form a recommenda-tion; the evidence needs to be interpreted. Box 3.5 lists the factors that contribute to deriving recommendations within a clinical practice guideline. Since conclusive evidence exists for few healthcare procedures, deriving recommendations solely in areas of strong evidence

Box 3.5. Factors contributing to the process of deriving recommendations

- the nature of the evidence (e.g. its susceptibility to bias)
- the applicability of the evidence to the population of interest (its generalisability)
- costs
- knowledge of the healthcare system
- beliefs and values of the panel.

would lead to a guideline of limited scope or applicability.[17] In certain limited circumstances, this could be sufficient if, for example, the guideline is to recommend the most strongly supported treatments for a given illness. More commonly the evidence needs to be interpreted into a clinical, public health policy or payment context. Therefore within the guideline development process a decision should be taken about how opinion will be both used and gathered.

Using and gathering opinion

Opinion will be used to both interpret evidence and derive recommendations in the absence of evidence. When interpreting evidence, opinion is needed to assess issues such as the generalisability of evidence. For example, opinion is needed to judge to what degree evidence from studies, such as small randomised clinical trials or controlled observational studies, may be generalised or to extrapolate results from a study in one population to the population of interest in the guideline (from a study in a tertiary, academic medical centre population to the community population of interest to potential users of the guideline).

Recommendations based solely on clinical judgement and experience are likely to be more susceptible to bias and self-interest. Therefore, after deciding what role expert opinion is to play, the next step is deciding how to collect and assess expert opinion. Unfortunately, less is known about how to assemble opinion sources than about how to collect and assess published literature, and there is no current gold standard method. Best practice is to at least make the process as explicit as possible.

Resource implications and feasibility

In addition to scientific evidence and the opinions of expert clinicians, practice guidelines must often take account of the resource implications and feasibility of interventions. Judgements about whether the costs of tests or treatments are reasonable depend on how cost effectiveness is defined and calculated, on the perspective taken (e.g. clinicians often view cost implications differently than would payers or society at large), and on the resource constraints of the healthcare system (e.g. cash-limited public versus private insurance-based systems). Feasibility issues worthy of consideration include the time, skills, personnel and equipment necessary for the provider to carry out the recommendations and the ability of patients and systems of care to implement them.

Grading recommendations

It is common to grade each guideline recommendation. Such information provides the user with an indication of the guideline development groups' confidence that following the guideline will produce the desired health outcome. While a number of 'strength of recommendation' classification schemes exist (see Box 3.4), from simple to complex, no classification scheme has been shown to be superior. However, given the factors that contribute to a recommendation (see Box 3.5), strong evidence does not always produce a strong recommendation and the classification should allow for this. The classification is probably best done by the group panel, using a democratic voting process after group discussion of the strength of the evidence.

External review of the guideline

Prior to finalising the guideline, we believe it is important to have external review of the guideline for content validity, clarity and applicability. External reviewers should cover three areas: 1) persons with clinical content expertise, who can review the guideline to verify the completeness of the literature review and to ensure clinical sensibility; 2) persons expert in systematic reviews and/or guideline development, who can review the method by which the guideline was developed; and 3) potential users of the guideline, who can judge the usefulness of the guideline. In the UK there is a further review process whereby guidelines are appraised by an independent unit to assess whether or not they can be commended by the NHS Executive to the NHS.

Updating of a guideline

This chapter has concentrated on the initial development of an evidence-based guideline. However, with time, new evidence will be published and should be incorporated into an updated version of the guideline. There are two potential ways of doing this. Either the guideline can be updated as soon as each and every piece of relevant new evidence is published, or a review date is specified in advance as the point at which the systematic review underpinning the guideline is updated. Because of the importance of the systematic review as the basis of the guideline and reflecting the need to identify all relevant evidence, we would argue that the latter is the better option. While experience with updating evidence-based guidelines is limited, the methods will be the same as in the initial development of the guideline and the resources required are likely to be of a similar magnitude.

Discussion

We have presented here a combination of the literature about guideline development and the results of our combined experience in guideline development in North America and Britain. The process of guideline development is dynamic, and it is likely that ongoing work on both sides of the Atlantic will expand the empirical evidence upon which our decisions about guideline development are based. New advances in understanding the science of systematic reviews, the workings of groups of experts, and the relationship between guideline development and implementation are all likely within the next three to five years.

We, however, believe that three principles will remain basic to the development of valid and useable guidelines: 1) the development of guidelines requires sufficient resources in terms of persons with a wide range of skills, including expert clinicians, health services researchers and group process leaders, and financial support; 2) a systematic review of the evidence should be at the heart of every guideline; and 3) the expert group assembled to translate the evidence into a guideline should be multidisciplinary.

Acknowledgement

During 1996 and 1997 Dr Shekelle was an Atlantic Fellow in Public Policy based at the National Primary Care Research and Development Centre in Manchester. Dr Shekelle is now a Research Associate of the Veterans Affairs Health Services Research and Development Service.

References

1 Woolf SH (1994) An organized analytic framework for practice guideline development: using the analytic logic as a guide for reviewing evidence, developing recommendations, and explaining the rationale. In: KA McCormick, SR Moore and RA Siegel (eds) *Methodology Perspectives*. US Department of Health and Human Services, Agency for Health Care Policy and Research, Washington, DC.
2 Kahan JP, Park RE, Leape LL *et al.* (1996) Variations by specialty in physician ratings of the appropriateness and necessity of indications for procedures. *Med Care* **34(6)**: 512–23.
3 Coulter I, Adams A and Shekelle P (1995) Impact of varying panel membership on ratings of appropriateness in consensus panels – a comparison of a multi- and single disciplinary panel. *Health Serv Res* **30(4)**: 577–91.
4 Leape LL, Park RE, Kahan JP and Brook RH (1992) Group judgments of appropriateness: the effect of panel composition. *Quality Assur Health Care* **4(2)**: 151–9.
5 Kosecoff JH, Kanouse DE, Rogers WH, McCloskey L,

Winslow CM and Brook RH (1987) Effects of the National Institutes of Health Consensus Development Program on physician practice. *JAMA* **258(19)**: 2780–93.

6 Shekelle PG and Schriger DL (1996) Evaluating the use of the appropriateness method in the Agency for Health Care Policy and Research Clinical Practice Guideline Development Process. *Health Serv Res* **31(4)**: 453–68.

7 Shekelle PG, Kravitz RL, Beart J, Morger M, Wang M and Lee M (2000) Are nonspecific practice guidelines potentially harmful? A randomized comparison of the effect of nonspecific or specific guidelines on physician decision making. *Health Service Research*. In press.

8 The Cochrane Library (2000) *The Cochrane Review Handbook*. Update Software, Oxford. In press.

9 Dickersin K, Scherer R and Lefebvre C (1994) Identifying relevant studies for systematic reviews. *BMJ* **309**: 1286.

10 Gregoire G, Derderian F and Le Lorier J (1995) Selecting the language of the publications included in a meta-analysis: is there a Tower of Babel bias? *J Clin Epidemiol* **48(1)**: 159–63.

11 Egger M, Zellweger-Zähner, Schneider M, Junker C, Lengeler C and Antes G (1997) Language bias in randomised controlled trials published in English and German. *Lancet* **350**: 326–9.

12 Strang N, Boissel JP and Uberla K (1997) Inter-reader variation. *5th Annual Cochrane Colloquium Abstract Book*: 279.

13 Colditz GA, Miller JN and Mosteller F (1989) How study design affects outcomes in comparisons of therapy, I: medical. *Stat Med* **8**: 441–54.

14 Miller JN, Colditz GA and Mosteller F (1989) How

study design affects outcomes in comparisons of therapy, II: surgical. *Stat Med* **8**: 455–66.

15 Schulz KF, Chalmers I, Hayes RJ and Altman DG (1995) Empirical evidence of bias: dimensions of methodological quality associated with estimates of treatment effects in controlled trials. *JAMA* **273(5)**: 408–12.

16 Moher D, Pham B, Jones A *et al.* (1998) Does quality of reports of randomised trials affect estimates of intervention efficacy reported in meta-analyses? *Lancet* **352**: 609–13.

17 Shekelle P, Chassin MR and Park RE (1998) Assessing the predictive validity of the RAND/UCLA appropriateness method criteria for performing carotid endarterectomy. *Int J Technol Assess Health Care* **14**: 707–27.

4

Clinical practice guidelines: legal, political and emotional considerations

Brian Hurwitz

Introduction

In the 4th century BC, Plato explored the difference between skills grounded in practical expertise and those based solely upon following instructions or obeying rules. Using the clinician as his model, he set up a thought experiment: doctors would be stripped of their clinical freedom – 'no longer allowed unchecked authority' – but would form themselves into councils to determine majority views about how to practise medicine in all situations.[1]

Plato's notion of codifying the majority decisions of

panels (composed of clinical and non-clinical members) and publishing their work, in order to influence (Plato says to dictate) 'the ways in which the treatment of the sick is practised', prefigures many of the impulses which animate the clinical guidelines movement today.

In Plato's view, important hallmarks of expertise include flexible responsiveness and 'improvisatory ability' – an approach to practice endangered, he believed, by use of guidelines. However effective health-care by guideline turned out to be – and Plato was prepared to concede its potential – it remained in his view a debased form of practice, because guidelines presuppose an average patient rather than the particular patient a doctor is endeavouring to treat, and because the knowledge and analysis that go into the creation of guidelines are not rooted in the mental processes of clinicians, but in the minds of guideline developers distant from the consultation. Similar concerns continue to trouble present-day clinicians (*see* Box 4.1).

Once the profession commits itself to providing health-

Box 4.1.

'There is a fear that in the absence of evidence clearly applicable to the case in hand a clinician might be forced by guidelines to make use of evidence which is only doubtfully relevant, generated perhaps in a different grouping of patients in another country and some other time and using a similar but not identical treatment. This is ... to use evidence in the manner of the fabled drunkard who searched under the street lamp for his door key because that is where the light was, even though he had dropped the key somewhere else.'[2]

care through guidelines (a position now demanded by government[3]), Plato could see no alternative but to ensure compliance with them, even if this entailed resorting to legal action. Such guidelines, he believed, have to be understood almost as clinical laws; for once expertise resides no longer within the patient's clinician but is represented in guidelines instead, corruption of or deviation from such guidelines would result in medical treatments being based on personal whim or quackery.

Plato's reference to the legal arena was remarkable in its prescience: only comparatively recently have guidelines begun to feature in healthcare regulations and case law.[4-8] That bias could creep into guideline development is a modern-day concern in France, where formal complaints have been laid before the Fraud Squad alleging improper conduct by participants in the French guidelines programme.[9]

Guidelines and legislation

Legislation in Europe and the USA has harnessed guidelines to a wide variety of regulatory tasks.[10,11] An example in the UK is the Human Fertilisation and Embryology Act 1990 which established a regulatory authority (HFEA) empowered to develop guidelines.[12] HFEA's decision to restrict to three the number of fertilised eggs which can be placed in a woman's uterus during treatment by in vitro fertilisation (IVF) is an example of a guideline that is unambiguously clear; and its mandatory nature in the event of transgression is made plain by enforceable penalties, including revocation of the licence to practise IVF. Though the guideline has been criticised as too restrictive, it nevertheless carries the force of a prescriptive legal rule; indeed, it has become almost an integral part of the legal framework itself (though HFEA retains the power to alter it).

In France, some 147 mandatory practice guidelines have been introduced under a 1993 statute, Loi Teulade 93–8, covering investigations, prescribing and certain medical procedures. Initially developed by the social security administration responsible for reimbursing private practitioners and the doctors' unions, guideline development has now been taken over by an independent organisation, the Agence Nationale pour le Développement de l'Évaluation Médicale. Once published, the guidelines constitute an enforceable agreement between doctors and the social security administration.[9,13]

Standards of medical care

The legally required standard of medical care a doctor generally owes to a patient derives in the UK from the case of *Bolam v Friern Hospital Management Committee* (1957). In the words of the judge in this case: 'The test is the standard of the ordinary skilled man exercising and professing to have that special skill.'[14] The judge recognised that there can be two or more schools of thought regarding proper medical treatment, so doctors can usually rebut a charge of negligence if they act in conformity with a body of other responsible doctors[14] (*see* Box 4.2).

Expert testimony helps the courts to ascertain what is accepted and proper practice in specific cases, ensuring that professionally generated standards from real clinical situations are generally applied, rather than standards enunciated in the rhetoric of clinical guidelines.[5] In

Box 4.2. Negligence

Medical negligence refers to a composite akin to a clinical syndrome comprising three essential elements.

A plaintiff – the person bringing the action – must show that:

- the defendant doctor owed the plaintiff a duty of care
- the doctor breached this duty of care by failing to provide the required standard of medical care
- this failure actually caused the plaintiff harm, a harm that should have been foreseeable and reasonably avoidable[15]

Clinical guidelines could, in theory, influence the manner in which the courts establish the second element of the syndrome.[16]

Cranley v Medical Board of Western Australia (1992) an Australian GP stood accused of misconduct because he had prescribed injectable diazepam to heroin addicts, contrary to the Australian National Methadone Guidelines. He was initially found guilty of 'infamous and improper conduct', but after hearing of a minority medical opinion supporting treatment of opiate addicts within the harm reduction framework followed by Dr Cranley, the Supreme Court of Western Australia upheld his appeal.[17]

The Bolam test, as a norm, is supposed to represent an aggregate of individual clinical judgements informed by scientific evidence and professional experience. Its advantages are that it takes account of evolving standards of care, and is a professionally lead, though legally imposed, standard. It allows for differences of opinion, and is sufficiently broadly expressed to encompass medical practice that is predominantly scientific or as much a craft as a science.

However, it appears to be a descriptive test about what is done in practice, rather than a normative one about what ought to be done. Widespread adoption of guidelines could therefore result in guideline-informed care becoming viewed as the customary norm. Departure from guidelines could then be seen as *prima facie* evidence of a case to answer.[18] The main justification for judicial reliance upon customary care standards has hitherto been the belief that medical technical matters are beyond the ken of judges and lay people, and are best left to 'experts'. Since guidelines offer doctors, patients and purchasers explicit examples of standards of care articulated in considerable detail for use in specific clinical circumstances, they could be thought to remove the need for expert testimony in court, as the courts would have direct access to relevant standards from guidelines (*see* Box 4.3).[19]

However, guidelines may not in fact reflect customary

Box 4.3.   Role of guidelines in court

Guidelines could be introduced to a court by an expert witness as evidence of accepted and customary standards of care, but they cannot be introduced as a substitute for expert testimony. Courts are unlikely to adopt standards of care advocated in clinical guidelines as legal 'gold standards', because the mere fact that a guideline exists does not of itself establish that compliance with it is reasonable in the circumstances, or that non-compliance is negligent.

standards of care at all. Indeed, some appear designed to hasten the incorporation of research findings into routine practice.[20] Adoption of a strong research and development strategy in the NHS which values rapid research implementation inevitably challenges the law's use of a customary care standard that does little to narrow gaps between everyday clinical practices and evidence-based practice. But though Bolam is clearly coming under pressure from a variety of sources, it appears unlikely to be superseded in the near future by a legal standard entirely determined without reference to a responsible body of medical practitioners.[15]

Author or sponsor liability

We have not found any UK common law cases in which the courts have had to consider whether authors of clinical guidelines could be liable for incorrect or misleading statements in circumstances where patients have suffered harm as a result.[16,21] In non-medical spheres, however, courts have decided similar questions where people have suffered economic loss by relying upon written statements of advice.[22]

There can be no duty of care between the author of a document or book and its myriad potential readers, unless the authors could foresee that their written advice would be directly communicated to a reader who would have little choice but to rely upon it without independent enquiry. Such advice would need to possess quite extraordinary authority for doctors to be expected to follow clinical guidelines without further inquiry (see Box 4.4).[23]

The legal status of guidelines could be made clear to clinicians if prefaced with statements such as that which

Box 4.4.   Author/sponsor liability[24]

'While an action could be taken against a clinician for not keeping up to date, a college is probably not actionable, as it would be difficult to show it owes a duty or obligation directly to the patient.'

introduces the 1997 guidelines for the prevention of malaria in travellers from the United Kingdom:

> *The views expressed in these guidelines reflect experienced professional opinion, since the data are inadequate for unequivocal views to be given on several issues. There is often a range of acceptable options ... Decisions on the terms under which different drugs are licensed for use are the responsibility of the Licensing Authority ... (not of these guidelines). The guidelines should be read as a supplement to and not as a substitute for the relevant data sheets.'[25]*

Though this reads like the disclaimer which it is clearly designed to be, the authors emphasise that guideline users are expected to behave as learned intermediaries, exercising customary clinical discretion and consulting other sources of relevant information.

Discretion

Clinicians fear that guideline proliferation will increase their medico-legal exposure,[26] but the only published study of actual guideline use in litigation revealed that guidelines play 'a relevant or pivotal role in the proof of negligence' in less than 7% of US malpractice actions.[27] Some health service lawyers have commented that as guidelines receive increasing acceptance in the clinical community, acting in accordance with a clinical guideline could be viewed as acceptable medical practice per se. However, a recent court case confirms there is currently no expectation, on the part of the courts, that guidance from works of reference with the standing of Martindale's Extra Pharmacopoeia or the British National Formulary should automatically be translated into clinical practice.[28] Doctors are expected to use appropriate clinical discretion, and the courts continue to place the testimony of expert witnesses about what constitutes reasonable practice above the recommendations of prestigious works of reference. Even where a guideline has been laid down as a legal standard, courts require that sensible discretion be used in its appropriate application.[29]

In administrative law the essence of discretion is 'a readiness to deal with each case on its merits.'[30] The NHS Executive acknowledges that when endorsed by prestigious professional bodies or even commended by the NHS Executive:

> 'clinical guidelines can still only assist the practitioner; they cannot be used to mandate, authorise or outlaw treatment options. Regardless of the strength of the evidence, it will remain the responsibility of the practising clinicians to interpret their application ... It would be wholly inappropriate for clinical guidelines to be used as a means of coercion of the individual clinician, by managers and senior professionals.'[31]

Rigid, uncritical adherence to guidelines is not the

formal, administrative or managerial expectation in the NHS. Though purchasers have been urged no longer to buy treatments but treatment protocols,[32] they need to recognise that translation of precepts into action involves interpretation,[33] as emphasised in guidelines on the treatment of hypertension produced by the World Health Organisation:

> 'Guidelines should provide extensive, critical, and well-balanced information on benefits and limitations of the various diagnostic and therapeutic interventions so that the physician may exert the most careful judgement in individual cases.'[34]

Concern remains, however, that guidelines will erode clinical abilities, diminish clinical judgement and reduce medical practice to 'cookbook medicine' and the thoughtless activities of physician automata.[35] In the USA, tensions surfacing between treatment protocols and doctors' clinical judgement have led the courts to rule that clinicians may not claim as a defence to negligence that their clinical judgement has been corrupted by guidelines.[36]

Although some judgements required of doctors in discrete areas of medicine can be more or less explicitly specified, this does not reduce clinical judgement to nothing other than 'decisional algebra' which can be objectified in expert systems, algorithms, protocols or guidelines. The routine reality of practice involves judgements about complex individual circumstances in the context of different degrees of uncertainty, where opinions differ, and where the authority of one's senses, perceptions and intuitions frequently play interacting roles.

Medical decision making involves making opinionated assessments which are grounded in knowledge of appropriate scientific findings, counterweighted by clinical experience and sensitive to patients' wishes. Such decisions are not simply transductions of input information resulting in output decisions. Clinical judgements frequently go beyond explicit input information, adding considerations of feeling, attitude and value to the output.[37] Researchers, health service managers and those involved in audit need to bear this complexity in mind when reporting wide variations in healthcare practices not accounted for by differences in patient case mix, or the circumstances of practice. Applying guidelines to individual care is always likely to require judgement, even when recommendations are properly evidence linked.[38]

Guidelines have an important role in addressing variation in healthcare standards, especially where there is strong evidence for effective treatment, and where significant departure from this occurs without valid justification. It is a mistake, however, to turn this argument round to maintain that clinical guidelines are required in order to remedy practice variation, without first studying why variations exist. Inherent uncertainties, lack of evidence, poor consensus, differences in patient choices and expectations may all underpin clinical practice variation.[37]

Conclusions

Sir Douglas Black envisages a time when 'the Pharisee and the reductionist might discover and explore dangerous common ground in a system of medical accountability based on a rule book, itself a compote of guidelines'.[39] But despite stirrings afoot to replace the customary standard of medical care with a standard determined without reference to a professional body of opinion, UK case law tends not to substantiate such fears. Guidelines are not credited by the courts with a special 'self-evident' status, and clinical guidelines currently play a subservient role to that of the expert witness in court proceedings. However, since guidelines are set to become more influential in both the way we practise and the manner in which we are to be held accountable, we need to pay attention to how we wish guideline and user to interact. If partnership between user and guideline is the preferred relationship, then we must create possibilities for productive dialogue between guideline developers and users.

We also need to know more about the cognitive processes involved in using guidelines actively and inter-actively, the sort of discretion that is exercised in their use, and how this may differ from that exercised in using other decision-making aids, such as textbooks, lecture notes or expert systems.

Officially, there may be no managerial or legal expectation that doctors should automatically follow guidelines, but purchasers may adopt a different view. Unlike the consensus guidelines of Plato, modern-day, evidence-linked clinical guidelines seek to make transparent the strengths, weaknesses and relevance of research findings to clinical care. Even where such guidelines are formulated as behavioural rules, their appropriate interpretation and application are likely to constitute better clinical care and a safer medico-legal strategy than uncritical disregard or unthinking compliance.[40]

References

1 Annas J and Waterfield R (eds) (1995) *Plato. Statesman.* Cambridge University Press, Cambridge (60–1).
2 Grimley Evans J (1995) Evidence-based and evidence-biased medicine. *Age and Ageing* **24**: 461–3.
3 Secretary of State for Health (1997) *The New NHS.* The Stationery Office, London.
4 Re F (Mental patient: sterilisation) (1989) *2 Weekly Law Reports* 1025–62.
5 Loveday v Renton and Wellcome Foundation Ltd (QBD) (1990) *1 Medical Law Reports* 117–204.
6 Re W (A minor) (1992) *3 Weekly Law Reports* 758–82.
7 Airedale NHS Trust v Bland (Guardian ad litem) (1993) *1 All England Reports* 821–96.
8 Early v Newham Health Authority (1994) *5 Medical Law Reports* 215–17.
9 Maisonneuve H, Codier H, Durocher A and Matillon Y (1997) The French clinical guidelines and medical references programme: development of 48 guidelines for private practice over a period of 18 months. *Journal of Evaluation in Clinical Practice* **3**: 3–13.
10 Ministry of Justice (1994) Directie Voorlichting: Act amending Act on the Disposal of the Dead. Staatsblad, 1993: 643. In: G van der Wal and RJ Dillman (1994) Euthanasia in the Netherlands. *BMJ* **308**: 1346–9.
11 Public Law 101–239, the Omnibus Reconciliation Act 1989. In: M Field and K Lohr (eds) (1990) *Clinical Practice Guidelines: directions for a new program.* National Academy Press, Washington. (107–27)
12 Human Fertilisation & Embryology Authority (1991) Code of Practice CH(91)5.

13 Durand-Zaleski I, Colin C and Blum-Boisgard C (1997) An attempt to save money using mandatory practice guidelines in France. *BMJ* **315**: 943–6.
14 Bolam v Friern Hospital Management Committee (1957) *2 All England Reports* 118–28.
15 Bolitho v City & Hackney Health Authority (1997) *3 Weekly Law Reports*: 1151–61.
16 Hurwitz B (1998) *Clinical Guidelines and the Law: negligence, discretion and judgment*. Radcliffe Medical Press, Oxford.
17 Cranley v Medical Board of Western Australia (Sup Ct WA) (1992) *3 Medical Law Reports* 94–113.
18 Harpwood V (1994) NHS reform, audit, protocols and standards of care. *Medical Law International* **1**: 241–59.
19 Stern K (1995) Clinical guidelines and negligence liability. In: M Deighan and S Hitch (eds) *Clinical Effectiveness: from guidelines to cost effective practice*. Earlybrave Publications Ltd, Brentwood.
20 Haines A and Jones R (1994) Implementing findings of research. *BMJ* **308**: 1488–92.
21 Newdick C (1995) *Who Should We Treat?* Clarendon Press, Oxford.
22 Caparo Industries plc v Dickman and others (1990) *1 All England Law Reports* 568–608.
23 National Health and Medical Research Council (1995) Legal implications of guidelines. In: *Guidelines for the Development and Implementation of Clinical Guidelines*. Australian Government Publishing Service, Canberra.
24 NHSE (1996) *Clinical Guidelines*. NHSE, Leeds.
25 Bradley DJ and Warhurst DC (1997) *Guidelines for the Prevention of Malaria in Travellers from the United Kingdom*. Communicable Disease Report, London.
26 Newton J, Knight D and Woolhead G (1996) General

practitioners and clinical guidelines: a survey of knowledge, use and beliefs. *Br J Gen Pract* **46**: 513–7.

27 Hyams AL, Brandenburg JA, Lipsitz SR, Shapiro DW and Brennan TA (1995) Practice guidelines and malpractice litigation: a two-way street. *Ann Inter Med* **122**: 450–5.

28 Vernon v Bloomsbury Health Authority (1995) *6 Medical Law Reports* 297–310.

29 McFarlane v Secretary of State for Scotland (1988) *Scottish Civil Law Reports* 623–8.

30 Cane P (1992) *An Introduction to Administrative Law.* Clarendon Press, Oxford.

31 NHSE (1996) *Clinical Guidelines.* NHSE, Leeds.

32 Williams A (1994) How should information on cost effectiveness influence clinical practice? In: T Delamothe (ed) *Outcomes into Clinical Practice.* BMJ Publishing Group, London.

33 Hawkins K (1992) *The Uses of Discretion.* Clarendon Press, Oxford.

34 Subcommittee of WHO/ISH Mild Hypertension Liaison Committee (1993) Summary of 1993 World Health Organisation-International Society of Hypertension guidelines for the management of mild hypertension. *BMJ* **307**: 1541–6.

35 Ellwood PM (1988) Outcomes management, a technology of patient experience. *NEJM* **318**: 1549–56.

36 Wickline v California (1996) *California Reporter* **228**: 661–67.

37 McPherson K (1990) Why do variations occur? In: TF Anderson and G Mooney (eds) *The Challenge of Medical Practice Variations.* Macmillan, London.

38 Black D (1998) The limitations of evidence. *J Roy Coll Phys* **32**: 23–5.

39 Black D (1998) Foreword. In: B Hurwitz *Clinical*

Guidelines and the Law: negligence, discretion and judgment. Radcliffe Medical Press, Oxford.

40 Dworkin R (1997) *Limits. The role of law in bioethical decision making.* Indiana University Press, Bloomington.

5

Using clinical guidelines

Gene Feder, Martin Eccles, Richard Grol, Chris Griffiths and *Jeremy Grimshaw*

Introduction

The development of good guidelines does not ensure their use in practice. Systematic reviews of professional behaviour-change strategies show that relatively passive methods of disseminating and implementing guidelines – by publication in professional journals or mailing to targeted healthcare professionals – rarely lead to changes in professional behaviour.[1,2] Lomas[3] observes that the failure of passive dissemination strategies is unsurprising, given that many factors influence healthcare professionals' behaviour. This has lead to increased recognition of potential barriers and facilitators to implementation at various levels: the organisation, the peer group and the individual clinician.

Therefore, to maximise the likelihood of a clinical guideline being used we need coherent dissemination and implementation strategies to capitalise on known facilitators and to address identified barriers. In this chapter, we discuss how healthcare organisations (e.g. hospitals, general practices) and individual clinicians can use clinical guidelines to improve clinical effectiveness. We suggest that there are two broad methods of effective guideline use, both of which should be planned, proactive processes. Firstly, healthcare organisations may use guidelines as tools within planned quality improvement activities; and secondly, individual healthcare professionals may use guidelines as an information source for continuing professional educational development and to answer specific clinical questions arising out of their day-to-day practice.[4,5]

Using clinical guidelines within healthcare organisations

The dissemination and implementation of guidelines as part of quality improvement activities within a healthcare organisation require planning, commitment, enthusiasm and resources. Quality improvement implies a cyclical process involving priority setting, implementation, assessment of performance (using clinical audit) and further implementation.

Preparation for dissemination and implementation

Priority setting

Healthcare organisations will only be able to support the implementation of a limited number of clinical guidelines at any one time. Therefore, in the same way as topics for guidelines development need to be prioritised,[6] organisations need a process by which they can set and pursue their clinical priorities. These can reflect national priorities or can be set at a local level by health authorities, trusts, primary care groups or individual general practices. Irrespective of the level at which priorities are set, explicit criteria can help guide a rational choice. A number of criteria for prioritising clinical topics have been suggested[7] and usually reflect considerations such as avoidable morbidity and mortality, inappropriate variation in performance, and health service expenditure. Such criteria then inform questions such as 'is there a problem in healthcare provision or in health outcomes (informed by the availability of audit data) and are there guidelines that cover this problem?'.

The nature of the healthcare organisation

When introducing clinical guidelines to improve patient care, a number of characteristics of the organisation will be important. At the simplest level the size and complexity of the organisation will affect the feasibility of different strategies. Strategies for a primary care group or a single-handed general practice may well be inappropriate in a large acute trust. For example, a strategy that involves face-to-face contact between a guidelines facilitator and all clinicians may be realistic for general practices but more difficult, if not impossible, within a large acute trust.

The culture of an organisation, specifically its approach and response to change, will also affect how guideline introduction should be approached. An organisation that has the ability to adapt to frequent change will offer different barriers and facilitators from one that is orientated towards maintaining the status quo.

Resources

The introduction of clinical guidelines requires resources. These include the costs of guidelines' production, but this is dwarfed by the time of appropriately skilled and experienced individuals who will conduct dissemination and implementation. At an organisational level the following skills are needed: knowledge of the theoretical basis of healthcare professional behaviour change and the empirical evidence about the effectiveness of different dissemination and implementation strategies;[2] good interpersonal skills; and knowledge of guideline development and appraisal methods. There may also be a need for specific skills for monitoring guidelines' use – data-processing skills for audit and feedback data or data collector skills for non-routine clinical data.

Finally, the introduction of guidelines will require the resources of clinicians within the organisation, to participate in prioritisation and guideline adaptation (see below) and also to use clinical guidelines in the care of patients. Ideally, the healthcare organisation needs to make a corporate decision to commit to these resources and to protect the time of individuals involved.

Finding valid guidelines to use

Most healthcare organisations do not have adequate resources and skills to develop valid guidelines de novo.[6,8] Instead, we recommend that healthcare organisations should attempt to identify previously developed rigorous guidelines and adapt these for local use.[8]

Identifying published guidelines

Identifying published clinical guidelines is problematic. Many guidelines are published in the grey literature and are not indexed in the commonly available bibliographic databases. There are a number of sources available, including sites on the Internet, that catalogue clinical guidelines (*see* Box 5.1). It is likely that such sites will become the best source to identify guidelines in the future, with an increasing number making full-text versions or abstracts of guidelines available.

If organisations cannot find published valid guidelines relevant to their identified priorities they face the choice of either amending their priorities or seeking to develop a guideline de novo. If they decide to develop a guideline, they should use as rigorous method as possible within the resources available[6] and be explicit about the development methods and their potential limitations. The increasing availability of high-quality systematic reviews in the Cochrane Database of Systematic Reviews

Box 5.1. Identifying guidelines

Search terms for common bibliographic databases

- Medline and Healthstar – *guideline* (publication type) and *consensus development conference* (publication type) (Note: Healthstar includes non-Medline referenced journals and grey literature, e.g. AHCPR guidelines).
- CINAHL – *practice guidelines* (publication type) (Note: Includes full-text version of some guidelines, including AHCPR guidelines).
- EMBASE – *practice guidelines* (subject heading) (Note: This is used for both articles about and which contain practice guidelines; furthermore the term was only introduced in 1994).

Useful websites

- Agency for Health Care Policy and Research guidelines – full-text versions of guidelines, quick reference guides and patient versions of guidelines can be downloaded from http://text.nlm.nih.gov/ftrs/dbaccess/ahcpr or ordered from the AHCPR website http://www.ahcpr.gov/cgi/bin/gilssrch.pl
- Canadian Medical Association Clinical Practice Guidelines Infobase – index of clinical practice guidelines, including downloadable full-text versions or abstracts for most guidelines (http://www.cma.ca/cpgs/index.html).
- Scottish Intercollegiate Guidelines Network – full-text versions of guidelines and quick reference guides (http://pc47.cee.hw.ac.uk/sign/home.htm).

and the Cochrane Controlled Trial Register (both available in the Cochrane Library[9]) makes this task slightly less daunting than previously.

Appraising guidelines

There are potential biases inherent in guideline development that need to be addressed to maximise the validity of the resulting guideline. When an organisation has identified relevant guidelines, it is important to appraise their validity before deciding whether to adopt their recommendations.[10] If organisations adopt recommendations from guidelines of questionable validity, this may lead to harm to patients or wasteful use of resources on ineffective interventions.[11] Within the United Kingdom, this task will be facilitated by the recently established NHS Appraisal Centre for Clinical Guidelines and by the establishment of guideline development programmes which use rigorous methods and include formal appraisal within the programmes (e.g. the Scottish Intercollegiate Guidelines Network[12] or the work proposed under the auspices of the National Institute for Clinical Excellence in England and Wales). If appraised guidelines are not available from these sources, organisations should undertake their own appraisal. A number of checklists for guideline appraisal have been proposed. Cluzeau and colleagues have developed and validated a critical appraisal tool for guidelines within UK settings[10] and other appraisal criteria are available.[13] We suggest that healthcare organisations should only consider guidelines that report development methods explicitly by including a methods section within the guideline or supporting papers.[14,15] Although using such a filter would exclude the majority of guidelines currently extant in the United Kingdom, without such information it is impossible to appraise the validity of guidelines and, as a result, difficult to have confidence in a guideline's recommendations.

Adaptation of valid guidelines

Once a group has identified guidelines of acceptable quality they need to be adapted for use within the local healthcare setting. The first step is setting up an appropriately multidisciplinary group. For most clinical conditions, good healthcare is dependent upon a multidisciplinary team, therefore guideline implementation should be planned from a multidisciplinary perspective. In terms of composition and function this group will parallel the original guideline development group[6] but will not need systematic reviewing and evidence-summarising skills. The task of the group is to adapt the guideline and then plan the presentation, use and evaluation of the guideline within the local setting. Adaptation of the guideline involves reformatting the guideline recommendations in terms of measurable criteria and targets for quality improvement.[5] This is particularly necessary given the general nature of most guidelines.

Two main factors will influence how a guideline is adapted by a local group: the strength of recommendation within the guidelines; and local circumstances. As a result of the subjective element involved in the interpretation of evidence when deriving recommendations, there is always the potential for a group to re-interpret evidence and derive different recommendations.

Deciding whether or not to derive different recommendations should be based, in large part, on the nature of the supporting evidence. Local adaptation groups should be wary of changing recommendations based upon good evidence, but may want to change recommendations based upon weak evidence. Where recommendations based on good evidence are changed the reasons for this should be explicitly stated.

In thinking about the use of the guideline the group will take account of specific local circumstances. The North of England Evidence-based Guideline on the use of ACE inhibitors in the management of patients with heart failure[16] suggests that, owing to the poor precision of clinical diagnosis, the diagnosis should be confirmed by echo cardiography. The local adaptation of this recommendation will be influenced by whether open-access facilities are available or whether access to echo cardiography is via a cardiologist.

A guideline adaptation group will then need to consider presentation, delivery, use and evaluation of the guideline as part of a coherent strategy.

Presentation

There will be a range of presentations from the full version of the guideline, summary sheets of all or part of the guideline, reminder sheets in patient records or various prompts such as guideline-related logos on mugs, pens or Post-It® pads. These strategies will overlap with use of the guideline when reminder sheets or computer templates are embedded within the patient record[17] or when test ordering forms are redesigned to encourage the gathering of appropriate clinical data.

Dissemination and implementation

Since there is no single effective way to ensure the use of guidelines in practice,[18-20] organisations should use multifaceted interventions to disseminate and implement guidelines. The choice of strategies should be informed by available resources, perceived barriers to care and research evidence about the effectiveness and efficiency of different strategies.[21] Systematic reviews of rigorous evaluations of dissemination and implementation strategies will provide the best evidence about their effectiveness and efficiency. Fortunately, there are an increasing number of systematic reviews of such strategies; in particular, the Cochrane Effective Practice and Organisation of Care group[2] undertakes systematic reviews of interventions designed to improve quality of care, including professional interventions (e.g. continuing medical education, audit and feedback, reminders), organisational interventions (e.g. the expanded role of pharmacists), financial interventions (e.g. professional incentives), and regulatory interventions.

There are a variety of potential professional and organisational strategies that address different barriers. For example, educational approaches (attendance at seminars and workshops) may be useful where barriers relate to healthcare professionals' knowledge. Audit and feedback may be useful when healthcare professionals are unaware of sub-optimal practice. Social influence approaches (local consensus processes, educational outreach, opinion leaders, marketing, etc.) may be useful when barriers relate to the existing culture, routines and practices of healthcare professionals. Reminders and patient-mediated interventions may be useful when healthcare professionals have problems processing information within consultations.

Information about existing barriers can be collected by interviews with individual patients or clinicians, group interviews or direct observation. The presence of organisational barriers may require specific interventions. For example, in east London, the development of primary care dyspepsia guidelines led to the commissioning of a direct-access *Helicobacter pylori* testing service for general practitioners.

Evaluation

Evaluation is important to ensure that the process of care reflects guideline recommendations. The necessary data to allow this should be specified at the outset and should be linked to areas of strong evidence within the guideline.[22] Reminder or prompt sheets can be designed to encourage the recording of specific data items.[17,23]

Medical or clinical audit advisory groups for general practice and clinical audit/clinical effectiveness departments in trusts have a key role to play in collecting, analysing and feeding back these data. Clinical governance – a central concept of the recent UK government's paper on the health service[24] – will depend on accurate and meaningful data about quality of care. We believe that criteria for clinical governance should be derived, at least in part, from the recommendations framed in evidence-based clinical guidelines.

Using guidelines for individual healthcare professionals

Outside a formal structure for the implementation of clinical guidelines within an organisation, individual clinicians may use guidelines as an information source for continuing professional education. Valid clinical guidelines provide an overview of the management of a condition or the use of an intervention. In this context, we argue that guidelines have potential advantages over systematic reviews. Guidelines usually have a broader scope than systematic reviews which tend to focus on an individual problem or intervention. They may also provide a more coherent integrated view on how to manage a condition. Guidelines can also be used as instruments for self-assessment or peer review to learn about gaps in performance. This is particularly relevant when the recommendations have been turned into specific measurable criteria.

Clinicians may also use guidelines to answer specific clinical questions arising out of their day-to-day practice. A key step is to frame the clinical question of interest in such a way that it can be answered specifying the patient or problem, the intervention of interest and possible comparison interventions and the outcomes of interest (*see* Sackett *et al.*[25] for a further discussion of this). This allows the clinician to identify what sort of evidence to search for. Under these circumstances clinical guidelines are only one of many types of evidence that are potentially relevant (systematic reviews; individual trials; expert advice).

Conclusions

Clinical guidelines are increasingly part of current practice and will become increasingly common over the next
decade. In this book we have suggested that great care
needs to be taken both to maximise the validity of guidelines and ensure use within clinical practice. The latter
requires adaptation for a local setting and the imagina-
tive use of evidence-based implementation strategies
tailored to relevant local factors. However, the implementation of clinical guidelines is not a panacea for all
the ailments of current clinical practice and should be
seen as only one of a number of potential strategies that
can help improve the quality of care that patients receive.

References

1 Freemantle N, Harvey E, Grimshaw JM, Wolf F, Bero
L, Grilli R and Oxman AD (1996) *The Effectiveness of
Printed Educational Materials in Changing the Behaviour
of Healthcare Professionals (Cochrane Review).* In: *The
Cochrane Library* (3e). Update Software, Oxford.
2 Bero L, Grilli R, Grimshaw JM and Oxman AD (eds)
(1998) *The Cochrane Effective Practice and Organisation
of Care Review Group. The Cochrane Database of Systematic Reviews* (2e). BMJ Publishing, London.
3 Lomas J (1994) Teaching old (and not so old) docs
new tricks: effective ways to implement research findings. In: EV Dunn, PG Norton, M Stewart, F Tudiver
and MJ Bass (eds) *Disseminating Research/Changing
Practice. Research Methods for Primary Care Volume 6.*
Sage Publications, Thousand Oaks.
4 Griffiths C and Feder G (1998) Using clinical guide-

lines in a general practitioner consultation. In: L Risdale (ed) *Evidence-based Practice in Primary Health Care*. Churchill Livingstone, London.

5 Grimshaw J and Eccles M (1998) Clinical practice guidelines. In: C Silagy and A Haines (eds) *Evidence-based Practice in Primary Care*. BMJ Publishing, London.

6 Shekelle PG, Woolf SH, Eccles M and Grimshaw J (1998) *Clinical Guidelines: developing guidelines*. BMJ Publishing, London.

7 NHS Executive (1996) *Clinical Guidelines: using clinical guidelines to improve patient care within the NHS*. NHSE, Leeds.

8 Royal College of General Practitioners (1996) *The Development and Implementation of Clinical Guidelines: report of the Clinical Guidelines Working Group. Report from Practice 26*. Royal College of General Practitioners, Exeter.

9 Cochrane Collaboration (1998) *The Cochrane Library* (3e). BMJ Publishing, London.

10 Cluzeau F, Littlejohns P and Grimshaw JM (1994) Appraising clinical guidelines – towards a 'Which' guide for purchasers. *Quality in Health Care* 3: 121–2.

11 Woolf SH, Grol R, Hutchinson A, Eccles M and Grimshaw J (1998) *Clinical Guidelines: the potential benefits, limitations, and harms of clinical guidelines*. BMJ Publishing, London.

12 Petrie JC, Grimshaw JM and Bryson A (1995) The Scottish Intercollegiate Guidelines Network initiative: getting validated guidelines into local practice. *Health Bulletin* **53**: 345–8.

13 Hayward RSA, Wilson MC, Tunis SR, Bass EB and Guyatt G (1995) Users' guides to the medical literature. VII. How to use clinical practice guidelines. A. Are the recommendations valid? *JAMA* **274:** 570–4.

14 Eccles MP, Clapp Z, Grimshaw JM, Adams PC, Higgins B, Purves I and Russell IT (1996) North of England evidence-based guideline development project: methods of guideline development. *BMJ* **312**: 760–1.

15 Eccles M, Freemantle N and Mason J (1998) Methods of developing guidelines for efficient drug use in primary care: North of England evidence-based guidelines development project. *BMJ* **316**: 1232–5.

16 Eccles M, Freemantle N and Mason J (1998) North of England Evidence-based Guidelines Development Project: evidence-based guideline for the use of ACE-inhibitors in the primary care management of adults with symptomatic heart failure. *BMJ* **316**: 1369–75.

17 Feder G, Griffiths C, Highton C, Eldridge S, Spence M and Southgate L (1995) Do clinical guidelines introduced with practice-based education improve care of asthmatic and diabetic patients? A randomised-controlled trial in general practices in east London. *BMJ* **311**: 1473–8.

18 Effective Health Care (1994) *Implementing Clinical Practice Guidelines*. **8**. University of Leeds, Leeds.

19 Oxman AD, Thomson MA, Davis DA *et al.* (1995) No magic bullets: a systematic review of 102 trials of interventions to improve professional practice. *Can Med Assoc J* **153**: 1423–31.

20 Wensing M and Grol R (1994) Single and combined strategies for implementing changes in primary care: a literature review. *Int J Qual Health Care* **6**: 115–32.

21 Grol R (1997) Beliefs and evidence in changing clinical practice. *BMJ* **315**: 418–21.

22 Agency for Health Care Policy and Research (1995) *Using Clinical Guidelines to Evaluate Quality of Care.*

Volume 1: Issues. US Dept of Health and Human Services, Public Health Service.

23 Emslie C, Grimshaw J and Templeton A (1993) Do clinical guidelines improve general practice management and referral of infertile couples? *BMJ* **306**: 1728–31.

24 NHS Executive (1998) *A First-class Service: quality in the new NHS.* NHSE, London.

25 Sackett DL, Richardson WS, Rosenberg W and Haynes RB (1996) *Evidence-based Medicine. How to practice & teach EBM.* Churchill Livingstone, New York.

6

Future developments for clinical guidelines

Martin Eccles and *Jeremy Grimshaw*

Introduction

The role of clinical guidelines within many healthcare systems has been given a new impetus from their inclusion as a central element of clinical effectiveness (*see* Chapter 2).[1,2] This has been influenced by the steadily accumulating body of evidence that guidelines can lead to improvements in both the process and outcome of care.[3,4]

This book has considered the current state of practice with relation to the need for guidelines, their development and use. However, the chapters pose as many questions as they answer. There is a need for greater knowledge regarding both the methods of development and the use of clinical practice guidelines. In this final chapter we highlight two areas within which such future developments may occur – the increasing sophistication of methods of guideline development, and an increased understanding of the factors that influence the implementation of guidelines, leading to methods for prioritising when to develop and implement guidelines.

Increasing the sophistication of guideline development methods

The guideline development process recognises the clinician–patient dyad as the decision-making unit. The role of the clinician is to gather sufficient data from the patient (from history or examination) to be able to make as confident a diagnosis as possible. She or he should then inform the patient about the potential management options and negotiate a management plan. These negotiations should be informed by patient, carer and clinician values and preferences, patient-specific information, the benefits, side-effects and safety of treatment and, to varying extents (depending perhaps on the mode of reimbursement), cost.

The role of a guideline is to support this negotiation by providing relevant information; consequently, the primary goal of guideline development is not to derive a single figure cost per quality-adjusted life-year, since this is the wrong form of presentation to inform such a doctor–patient interaction. Rather the objective is to help the clinician and patient together to perform appropriate aggregation of attributes of treatment and the weighing up of their relative importance in an individual treatment decision.

Types of evidence

The guideline process summarises the research evidence of treatments in a manner that makes them accessible and ready for use alongside contextual issues. The technical presentation requires the assessment of costs and benefits of treatment to be methodologically sound. However, most clinical guideline development has drawn almost exclusively on evidence of clinical effectiveness alone. There are clearly other dimensions of evidence that could reasonably be expected to influence the recommendations made by a guideline development group. While the introduction of broader dimensions of evidence generally[5,6] and cost considerations specifically[7]

Box 6.1. Issues to be addressed in clinical guidelines

- What evidence suggests that the services are likely to affect outcomes for the condition or intervention being considered?
- What groups at risk are most likely to experience benefits or harms from the proposed course of care and its side-effects?
- What is known about the effects of different frequencies, duration, dosages or other variations in the intensity of the intervention?
- What options in the ways services are organised and provided can affect the benefits, harms and costs of services?
- What benefits, harms and costs can be expected from alternative diagnostic or treatment paths, including watchful waiting or no intervention?

within guidelines has been argued for, it is unclear how the introduction of such data would influence the recommendations produced by a guideline development group.

The Committee on Clinical Practice Guidelines[6] recommended that every set of clinical practice guidelines include information from a range of evidence sources on the implications of alternative preventive, diagnostic, and management strategies for the clinical situation in question. Their stated rationale was that this information can help potential users to better evaluate the potential consequences of different practices. However, they aver that 'the reality is that this recommendation poses major methodological and practical challenges'. There is thus a mismatch between the need and the ability to do this. They suggest that in the process of considering these issues five theoretical questions should be considered (*see* Box 6.1); unfortunately the answers to these questions are problematic for a number of reasons (*see* Box 6.2).

Box 6.2.   Problems confronting guideline developers

- Scientific evidence about benefits and harms is incomplete.
- Basic, accurate cost data are scarce for the great majority of clinical conditions and services.
- While data on charges may be available, significant analytic steps and assumptions are required to treat charge data as cost data.
- Techniques for analysing and projecting costs and cost effectiveness are complex and only evolving.

Considering costs

The reasons for considering costs are clearly stated by Eddy:[5]

> 'Health interventions are not free, people are not infinitely rich, and the budgets of (healthcare) programmes are limited. For every dollar's worth of healthcare that is consumed, a dollar will be paid. Furthermore, the costs will be paid by present and future patients ... Such costs will be paid through insurance premiums, smaller employee benefit packages, lower salaries, the cost of commodities (cars, houses) or direct or indirect taxation. While these payments can be laundered, disguised or hidden, they will not go away. Therefore, the costs of interventions should be balanced against the health outcomes predicted for that intervention for two reasons. Firstly, at the level of individual patients, failure to make the comparison may cause people to receive (and thus pay for) interventions that they might otherwise have declined, had they been fully informed. Secondly, at the level of healthcare systems, costs must be considered if the available resources are to be used efficiently; failure to do this lowers the quality of care and harms the health of patients.'

Even having considered cost data in the light of these questions and limitations there is then the further question of how to use the data. Should it be presented alongside recommendations based solely on clinical effectiveness or should it be incorporated into the judgement process of deriving recommendations? Williams argues that guidelines based on effectiveness issues and then costed may differ substantially from and may be less efficient than guidelines based on cost-effectiveness issues.[7] The complexity of this process, and the reactions that it evokes are reflected by the Committee on Clinical Practice Guidelines report of 'much debate, and with some vigorous dissent'.[6] There is no widely accepted successful way to incorporate economic considerations into guidelines. Furthermore, given the prominence paid to systematic reviewing and evidence-based guideline construction it is unclear how 'evidence' from the methodology of health economics, with its reliance on modelling and assumption, will sit alongside 'evidence' derived from the rigour of systematic review.[8]

It is not clear how healthcare professionals will react to this process as most healthcare professionals have a limited knowledge of health economics and its methods. Guidelines based on clinical effectiveness could be enhanced or undermined by the incorporation of economic considerations, depending on whether they are seen as attempts to achieve cost-effectiveness or cost-containment. However, the incorporation of a wider range of evidence will begin to change the nature of the decision-making process within guideline groups. In the development of a guideline for the use of first-line antidepressants for the treatment of depression in UK primary care, the guideline development group had available a range of evidence about the two major drug groups.[9] The evidence showed no demonstrable difference in efficacy, no clinical (although a small statistical) difference in tolerability, large differences in drug acquisition costs and large differences in toxicity in overdose. The guideline development group found their decision being made not on considerations of efficacy but on the cost consequences of avoiding drug overdose-related deaths.

Finally, it is uncertain how the incorporation of economic considerations will affect the use of guidelines with individual patients. It will encourage a more explicit consideration of cost consequences both in determining available treatment options within a healthcare system and within consultations where a guideline is used. This is not a process that policy makers or health professionals are used to doing at anything other than an implicit level. However, the absence of economic data from guidelines may severely limit their usefulness to policy makers, clinicians and patients.

Understanding factors that influence the implementation of guidelines

Although there is increasing knowledge about methods of implementing guidelines, systematic reviews frequently find it difficult to offer firm conclusions due to: the complexity of behaviour change, and the large number of factors influencing intervention effectiveness; the limited number of studies available; limitations in the design of interventions; and limitations in the design and analysis of studies.[10–12] This means that healthcare professionals, policy makers and researchers have a relatively poor scientific basis on which to select strategies to implement guidelines in line with research findings. Increasingly clinical effectiveness programmes are being established in healthcare settings; however, within such programmes the choice of strategies to implement guidelines is often based on personal beliefs rather than evidence.[13]

Theories of behaviour, based on the cumulative evidence of research in social and behavioural sciences, are currently being used in only a limited way in implementation research. Theory has been invoked in a general way,[14,15] offering a descriptive framework which limits its value for those planning interventions. Interventions have been designed which social and cognitive theories[16] would suggest would be effective only in motivated populations (e.g. audit and feedback) and there has been subsequent disappointment at the limited effects. Recent reviews of implementation studies[17] suggested that few, if any, had an explicit theoretical base for their interventions and the results of the reviews could support a number of differing theoretical perspectives.[18]

Over the past five years there has been a considerable interest in evidence-based healthcare, with its emphasis on the appropriate identification of evidence to inform clinical practice. There has also been a considerable amount of empirically driven implementation research that demonstrates that, within the context of evaluative studies, it is possible to change healthcare professional behaviour.[8] Additionally, over the past decade there have been a number of professional and policy initiatives to promote uptake of research findings and improve quality of care (e.g. RCGP Quality Initiative[19], the PACE Programme[20], and clinical governance[2]).

However, such initiatives have not necessarily fully utilised the early findings of implementation research, and the extent to which they did or can achieve their policy objectives is uncertain. If clinical governance and related initiatives are to achieve their stated objectives it is important that policy decisions are based upon both the available findings of empirical guideline implementation research and appropriate theory to optimise the design and choice of interventions.

The goal in this area would be to move towards

having, on the basis of both theory and empirical evidence, a taxonomy that defines characteristics of settings, clinicians, patients, clinical activities and interventions and guides the choice of one or more optimum strategies for given circumstances. Such a taxonomy is currently available in only the most embryonic of forms.[4,10,12]

Prioritising when to develop and implement guidelines

Currently guidelines have been developed for many conditions with little underlying view on the appropriateness for their development. Ideally, guideline development and implementation should only be undertaken when this would lead to an efficient use of resources. However, there is little information about the general efficiency of guidelines and how this might vary, for example, across different settings, different targeted groups and clinical activities, and different development, dissemination and implementation strategies. Reviews of guideline development[21] and implementation have not explicitly addressed economic issues – in particular issues such as the incremental costs and benefits associated with different development dissemination and implementation strategies in different contexts and for different clinical problems. As a result, policy makers and clinicians have little to guide them about when it would be worthwhile to devote resources to guideline development and introduction for specific clinical problems.

However, with increasingly explicit criteria for the development of clinical guidelines and clear empirical evidence on the achievable benefits, it should be feasible to establish a set of quantifiable criteria which set out the likely cost effectiveness of developing guidelines. These could include the mismatch between current and optimum behaviour, the nature (including costs) of the activity (e.g. prescribing, performance of a screening procedure), the costs involved in developing an evidence-based guideline, and the cost effectiveness of available implementation strategies. Armed with such information policy makers would have a far more rational basis on which to prioritise guideline development and implementation.

Conclusions

Currently decisions have to be made in the face of imperfect evidence about how to best improve patient care with guidelines. As the methods of guideline development improve and understanding about how and when to implement guidelines develops we can look forward to having improved clinical guidelines and an improved basis on which to use them. However, it will remain the case that guidelines are not, and will almost certainly never be the panacea for all quality assurance ills. They will remain only one of the tools (albeit an increasingly sophisticated one) in the range of appropriate strategies to improve patient care.

References

1 NHS Executive (1996) *Clinical Guidelines: using clinical guidelines to improve patient care within the NHS.* The Stationery Office, London.

2 Department of Health (1997) *The New NHS: modern, dependable*. Department of Health, London.

3 Centre for Reviews and Dissemination and Nuffield Institute for Health (1994) Implementing clinical practice guidelines: can guidelines be used to improve clinical practice? *Effect Health Care* 1–12.

4 Centre for Reviews and Dissemination (1999) Getting evidence into practice. *Effect Health Care* **5**: 1–16.

5 Eddy DM (1992) *A Manual for Assessing Health Practices and Designing Practice Policies: the explicit approach*. American College of Physicians, Philadelphia.

6 Field MJ and Lohr KN (eds) (1992) *Guidelines for Clinical Practice: from development to use*. National Academy Press, Washington DC.

7 Williams A (1995) How should information on cost effectiveness influence clinical practice? In: T Delamothe (ed) *Outcomes into Clinical Practice* (1e). BMJ Books, London.

8 Grimshaw J, Eccles M and Russell I (1995) Developing clinically valid practice guidelines. *J Eval Clin Pract* **1**: 37–48.

9 Eccles M, Freemantle N and Mason JM (1999) The choice of antidepressants for depression in primary care. *Fam Pract* **16**: 103–11.

10 Bero L, Grilli R, Grimshaw JM, Harvey E, Oxman AD and Thomson MA (1998) Closing the gap between research and practice: an overview of systematic reviews of interventions to promote implementation of research findings by healthcare professionals. *BMJ* **317**: 465–8.

11 Oxman AD, Thomson MA, Davis DA and Haynes B (1995) No magic bullets: a systematic review of 102 trials of interventions to improve professional practice. *Can Med Assoc J* **153**: 1423–31.

12 Grimshaw J and Eccles M (1998) Clinical practice guidelines. In: C Silagy and A Haines (eds) *Evidence-based Practice in Primary Care*. BMJ Books, London.
13 Grol R (1997) Beliefs and evidence in changing clinical practice. *BMJ* **315**: 418–21.
14 Lomas J (1994) Teaching old (and not so old) docs new tricks: effective ways to implement research findings. In: EV Dunn, PG Norton, M Stewart, F Tudiver and MJ Bass (eds) *Disseminating Research/Changing Practice*. Sage, London.
15 Grol R (1992) Implementing guidelines in general practice care. *QHC* **2(1)**: 184–91.
16 Conner M and Norman P (1998) Health behaviour. In: DW Johnston and M Johnston (eds) *Health Psychology*. Elsevier, Oxford.
17 Solomon DH, Hashimoto H, Daltroy L and Liang MH (1998) Techniques to improve physician's use of diagnostic tests. *JAMA* **280**: 2020–7.
18 Davis DA, Thomson MA, Oxman AD and Haynes RB (1995) Changing physician performance: a systematic review of the effect of continuing medical education strategies. *JAMA* **274**: 700–5.
19 Royal College of General Practitioners (1985) *Quality in General Practice. Policy Statement 2*. RCGP, London.
20 Dunning M, Abi-Aad G, Gilbert D, Hutton H and Brown C (1999) *Experience, Evidence and Everyday Practice. Creating systems for delivering effective health care*. King's Fund, London.
21 Grimshaw JM, Freemantle N, Wallace S, Russell IT, Hurwitz B, Watt I, Long A and Sheldon T (1995) Development and implementation of clinical practice guidelines. *QHC* **4**: 55–66.

Index

Dutch College of General
Practitioners 33

economic implications 27
educational approaches 94
effectiveness, database of
abstracts of reviews of 57
EMBASE 57, *90*
England 32–3
Europe 32–6
European Union 35
evaluation of clinical guidelines
in use 95
evidence
developing guidelines *see*
developing guidelines
lacking 24
misinterpreted 24
misleading 24
types 103–7
evidence-based centres 36
evidence-based guidelines 22–3,
32–3
evidence-based healthcare 108
evidence-based methods 37, 38
expert opinion 32
expert testimony 72–3, 77
external review of guidelines 63

factors contributing to
recommendations *60*
FACTS (Framework for
Appropriate Care
Throughout Sheffield) 32
feasibility of recommendations
62
finding guidelines to use 89–91
Finland 34
flawed guidelines 25, 26

Framework for Appropriate
Care Throughout Sheffield
(FACTS) 32
France 34–5, 71, 72
future developments 101–2
development
cost considerations 105–7
evidence types 103–7
methods, increasing
sophistication 102–7
prioritising 109–10
implementation
prioritising 109–10
understanding factors
influencing 107–9

Germany 35
governance, clinical 95, 108
grading recommendations 62–3
guideline development groups
see developing guidelines
guidelines on guidelines 37

harms
to healthcare professionals
26–7
to healthcare systems 27–8
to patients 25–6
health outcomes, improvement
20
healthcare organisations
disseminating and using
clinical guidelines in 87–9
healthcare professionals
benefits for 22–3
harms to 26–7
using clinical guidelines 96
healthcare systems
benefits for 23–4

adaptation of valid guidelines
    92–3
  dissemination and
      implementation 94–5
  evaluation 95
  presentation 93
appraising guidelines 91–2
audit advisory groups 95
audit and feedback 94
clinical questions in day-to-
    day practice 96
educational approaches 94
finding guidelines to use 89
  identifying published
      guidelines 89–91, 90
in healthcare organisations 86
  nature of organisation 87–8
  preparation 87–9
  priority setting 87
  resources 88–9
individual healthcare
    professionals 96

multidisciplinary teams 92
patient-mediated
    interventions 94–5
as peer review instruments
    96
professional behaviour-
    change 85–6
prompt sheets 95
quality improvement
    activities 86
reminders 94–5
as self-assessment instruments
    96
social influence approaches
    94

value judgements 24

websites 90
World Health Organisation
    (WHO)
  guidance on guidelines 78